Substance misuse in pregnancy

A resource book for professionals

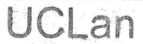

Substance misuse in pregnancy

A resource book for professionals

Published by
DrugScope
32 Loman Street
London SE1 OEE
Tel 020 7928 1211
Fax 020 7928 1771
E-mail: info@drugscope.org.uk
Website: www.drugscope.org.uk

First published by NHS Lothian 2003
This edition DrugScope 2005

ISBN 1904319 351
Design: Andrew Haig Associates
Printed in Great Britain by College Hill Press

DrugScope has a range of products and services for practitioners
and policymakers. For further information, please visit our website
or contact us for a catalogue.

Enquirers may contact the Information service by phone, letter fax or email.
Enquiry line: 08707 743 682 Monday to Friday 10am to 1pm
Email: info@drugscope.org.uk
Written enquiries: Information & Library Service, DrugScope,
32 Loman Street SE1 OEE

The Library is open for research, by appointment only, Monday to Friday,
hours by arrangement

Acknowledgements for the original edition

Many professionals contributed to, supported and offered constructive suggestions and comments on the numerous drafts of this resource pack. The professional groups from Lothian who contributed to the pack include: midwives, maternity and neonate nurses, obstetricians and gynaecologists, neonatologists and paediatricians, health visitors, general practitioners, pharmacists, drug specialists, alcohol specialists, HIV specialists, public health staff, dental hospital staff, social work and voluntary sector staff.

Anne would like to thank the following people: Pauline Connolly, Fiona McGuckin, Fiona McNeilage, Mary Simpson and all the Link Midwives for Substance Misuse, Chris Vinestock, Julia Holmes, Maria Wilson, Karla Napier, Agnes Moretta, Susan Stewart, Frances McGuire, Doreen Trainor, Dr Rhona Hughes, Dr Wang Liston, Dr Gerry Beattie, Dr Paula Midgley, Dr Jacqueline Mok, Dr Helen Hammond, Dr Karen Barclay, Jenny Carson, Sherry Wright, Alison Conlon, Dr Gordon Scott, Dr Fiona Watson, Dr Malcolm Bruce, Dr David Miles, Dr Catriona Morton, Dr Roy Robertson, Dr Muriel Simmonte, Jim Shanley, Jim Sherval, Dr Margaret Douglas, Graham Lyell, John Vevers, Jane Todd, Dr Judy Bury, Rosina Weightman, Dr Ewen Stewart, Dr David Ewart, Dr Jonathan Chick, Dr Claire McIntosh, Barbara McKenzie, Louise Learmonth, Karen Thorburn, Gail Trotter, Dee Mills, Jane Henry, Chris Cunningham, Ray deSouza, Geraldine Brown, Bertie Goffe, Brian Pringle, Claire Thomas, Liz Dahl and Dr Mary Hepburn.

Anne would especially like to thank Patricia Drake who provided invaluable administrative and secretarial support.

Finally, a special thanks to all the service users who contributed to the development of the service user information leaflets.

About this new DrugScope edition

The original text was written by Anne Whittaker and first published by NHS Lothian in 2003. Much of this text has been retained. However, we have tried to ensure that the material is now more relevant to the wider UK audience. This means, for example, we have removed references to local services in Lothian and made some changes (e.g. on prescribing) to reflect wider UK practice. The Appendices are largely as originally published, but are included as useful templates which can be adapted by any service.

Contents

Introduction 7

Key points 8

Setting the scene 11

  The extent of the problem 11

  The nature of the problem 11

    Organisational difficulties 12

    Ideology 12

    Research evidence 13

    Women's fears 13

    Poor social circumstances 13

    Maternal health problems 14

    Chaotic lifestyle 14

    Obstetric and paediatric problems 14

Framework for care 16

  Philosophy of approach 16

    Women and family centred approach 16

    Non-judgemental approach 17

    Harm reduction approach 18

    Holistic approach 18

    Multi-disciplinary and multi-agency approach 19

Guidelines on good practice 20

  The care process 20

    Assessment 20

    Care planning 22

    Reviewing the care plan 23

    Care management 23

    Consent to share information 24

Information and guidelines on drug use 25

  Trends in substance use 25

  Effects of commonly used drugs 25

  Injecting drug use 27

Drugs and their effects on the developing baby 28

  Evidence base 29

    Effects of tobacco 29

    Effects of alcohol 30

    Effects of drugs (illicit and prescribed) 31

Neonatal Abstinence Syndrome (NAS) 35
Signs and symptoms of NAS 35
Assessment of NAS 37
Preparing parents for NAS 38
Management of neonatal withdrawal symptoms 38
Management of substance use in pregnancy 42
Smoking cessation 42
Advice on alcohol consumption 43
Antenatal screening for problem drinking 44
Management of problem alcohol use 45
Alcohol detoxification 46
Assessing drug related problems 47
Management of problem drug use 47
Safer drug use 48
Substitute prescribing 48
Stabilisation 50
Reduction 51
Detoxification 52
Maternity care 53
Pre-conception care 53
Reproductive health and drug use 53
Pre-conception advice 54
Antenatal care 56
Hand held maternity records 57
The booking appointment 57
Routine antenatal screening at booking 58
Other screening and diagnostic tests 58
Pregnancy complications 60
Maternal health problems 60
Benefits and allowances 61
Preparation for parenthood 61
Risk assessment during pregnancy 62
Homelessness 62
Not registered with a GP 63
Domestic abuse 63
Neonate at risk of NAS 63
Child care risk 64

Intrapartum care (labour and childbirth) 65

Maternity hospital policy 65

Pain relief during childbirth 66

Complications of childbirth 66

Postpartum care in hospital 67

Infant feeding 70

Breastfeeding 70

Weaning 71

Bottle feeding 72

Postnatal care 72

Postnatal depression 73

Sudden Infant Death Syndrome (SIDS) 73

Risk of relapse 73

Assessing and managing child care risk during pregnancy 75

Child protection 77

Early intervention strategies 78

Protective factors 78

Service providers 80

References 83

Glossary 88

Appendices

1. Blood Borne Viruses 92

2. Model Care Pathway 101

3. Consent form for multi-disciplinary working 104

4. GP allocation proforma letter 106

5. T-ACE alcohol screening questionnaire 107

6. TWEAK alcohol screening questionnaire 108

7. Drug and Alcohol Diary 109

8. Midwifery Liaison Forms (Substance Misuse) 110

9. NAS assessment score chart 116

10. Leaflet: *Pregnant ... and using alcohol and drugs?* 118

11. Leaflet: *Caring for a baby with drug withdrawal symptoms* 125

Introduction

Many different professionals and service providers are now involved in the care of women who use drugs and/or alcohol during the course of their reproductive life. All professionals have an equally important role to play in ensuring a high standard of care is delivered. *Substance misuse in pregnancy* aims to establish a 'framework for care' so that all women who use drugs can be offered appropriate support before, during and after the birth of their child.

A broad view of drug use is taken that includes *alcohol* and *nicotine*. This is because the risks of these drugs in pregnancy are well established and they are often used in combination with illicit and prescribed drugs.[1] Having said this, the book refers mainly to the care of women who have *significant* problems related to drug and alcohol use. This is because *social and lifestyle factors* often complicate the delivery of care to these women. Their care often provides the biggest challenge for professionals and much co-ordination and understanding between services is needed.

The terminology used has been carefully chosen so as to avoid language that implies value judgements or has negative connotations. For instance, the terms *drug and alcohol dependency, drug and alcohol related problems, drug use* or *substance misuse* are used in preference to terms such as *addiction, drug addict, alcoholic, drug habit* or *drug abuse*. The use of currently preferred terminology is especially important when working with substance-misusing women who are particularly sensitive to public and professional judgements.

The information and advice is based on current *best practice* and available *evidence*. Sources include: governmental policy documents, contemporary social theory and health care practice, good practice guidelines, expert opinion and recent publications from experienced practitioners in the field as well as a literature and publications search.

The book is not fully referenced but those references that are cited are recommended for further reading. Other helpful sources of information, addresses and websites are included. A glossary provides definitions of terms.

The book is not designed to be read cover to cover but it is worth taking a little time to familiarise yourself with the layout and contents so that you can access information easily when you need to. It is worthwhile reading the 'key points' and 'philosophy of approach' before other sections.

---

1. *Johnstone 1998.*

Key Points

- Most pregnant women with substance misuse problems will have a normal pregnancy, labour, delivery and a full-term normal birth-weight baby. Most will embrace motherhood and cope well with caring for their children.

- Many conditions carry with them an element of risk or uncertainty during pregnancy and require greater care. Increased risks are associated with smoking, alcohol use and drug use in pregnancy. Agencies should work together to offer information, advice, treatment and care that will help reduce these risks.

Philosophy of approach

- Many factors affect pregnancy outcome and the health and development of infants and children. Substance misuse is just one factor. A holistic assessment and package of care needs to be offered. The woman's lifestyle and social circumstances, her physical and psychological needs, her support needs, as well as the needs of her unborn child should be taken into account.

- The approach taken by professionals is a crucial factor in the delivery and outcome of care. Pregnant women with substance misuse problems are subject to social disapproval and judgemental attitudes. Discriminatory professional practice deters women from seeking help. Professionals need to encourage women to engage with helping agencies and ensure that their approach to care is based on good evidence and best practice.

- The guiding principle of management should be a pragmatic approach that emphasises harm reduction and aims to achieve the best possible outcome for both mother and baby. This means taking account of the woman's wishes, recognising her vulnerabilities and needs and focusing on what *could* be done rather than what *should* be done.

- A well co-ordinated multi-disciplinary and multi-agency approach will ensure that a comprehensive package of care can be offered. All professionals involved in a woman's care need to communicate with one another to ensure that they share a common approach, offer consistent advice and are working towards the same goals.

Pre-conception care

- Agencies in contact with substance-misusing women should routinely enquire if they plan to have children. All agencies have a part to play in offering pre-conception advice and care.

Antenatal care

- All pregnant women with substance misuse problems and their partners should be told about the benefits of antenatal care and encouraged to attend early in pregnancy.

- Specific information and advice about the effects of drug use (including tobacco and alcohol) on pregnancy should be routinely given to all women identified as having a substance misuse problem.

- Drug dependent women should be given information and advice on Neonatal Abstinence Syndrome (NAS) and helped to prepare for the care of their newborn baby.

- Pregnant women and their partners should be given priority access to drug and alcohol treatment services. Treatment goals should be realistic and tailored to their individual needs.

Assessing risk in pregnancy

- Professionals should undertake a continuous risk assessment throughout pregnancy to identify any problems that could affect the mother, her pregnancy and the well being of the baby.

- Substance misuse is not sufficient reason in itself, to assume that parenting or childcare will be inadequate. However, the safety and welfare of the newborn baby is paramount and professionals should follow child protection guidelines if 'significant harm' is likely.

Intrapartum care

- Although most women with substance misuse problems will have a normal labour and delivery, they may need help to prepare for hospital admission. Drug dependent women should be reassured that they will be given adequate pain relief during childbirth.

● Following delivery, parents should care for their baby as normal in the postnatal ward. Separating mother and baby should be avoided wherever possible. Like other women, they should be encouraged to breastfeed, bond and care for their baby.

Postnatal care

● Parents with substance misuse problems may need considerable help and support to cope with the transition into parenthood. Planned support that continues into the postnatal period is crucial.

● The postnatal period can be a stressful time for parents. For mothers who have managed to reduce their drug and alcohol use during pregnancy, the risk of relapse to former levels of drug taking is high. Relapse prevention work, careful drug management and intensive psychosocial support may be required for some time.

Setting the scene

The extent of the problem

The true extent of drug taking in women is largely unknown as reliable figures are hard to obtain. It is clear, however, that smoking, alcohol use and illicit drug use in women of reproductive age is increasing and the continued use of drugs during pregnancy is common. Approximately one-third of pregnant women smoke and approximately 60 per cent continue to consume alcohol.[2] The use of illicit drugs in pregnancy such as cannabis, amphetamines, heroin and cocaine is thought to be fairly widespread, especially in large urban areas. For many women, drug use is a 'lifestyle choice' and a fundamental part of their lives.

Although nicotine and alcohol are legally available it is important not to confuse **legality** with **safety**. Maternal use of tobacco is well researched and known to have significant harmful effects on pregnancy. Although approximately 25 per cent of women who smoke manage to give up during pregnancy, nicotine remains the most problematic drug of use in pregnancy at a population level.[3] Alcohol has the clearest association with *teratogenesis* (congenital birth defects), with well-documented adverse effects associated with high maternal intake. Approximately 20 per cent of women of reproductive age exceed the recommended weekly limit of alcohol consumption. Nicotine and alcohol are often used in combination with other drugs and most women who present to drug and alcohol treatment services report *polydrug use.*

The nature of the problem

Many factors affect the outcome of pregnancy and the health and well being of mother and baby. Many conditions carry with them an element of risk or uncertainty and require greater care during pregnancy. Drug use is just one factor. Other factors include lifestyle and social circumstances, physical and psychological health, nutrition, breastfeeding, sexually transmitted and communicable diseases, antenatal and postnatal care.

Women who seek help for drug and alcohol related problems are more likely to be unemployed and living in areas of *social deprivation.* Pregnant women with substance misuse problems often present with a *multiplicity of needs* that require the involvement of many different professionals and agencies. The *organisation* and *delivery* of care therefore, is an important factor in outcome.

---

2. *Taylor 2003*
3. *Johnstone 1998*

Organisational difficulties

Professionals who are experienced in working with this client group often report a number of problems. These include:
- No common or 'shared' approach to care
- Lack of understanding of professional roles and responsibilities
- Poor liaison and communication between professionals
- Little consultation or 'joint' assessments
- Limited 'partnership' of care with the woman
- Unrealistic expectations and treatment goals
- Inconsistent and contradictory advice
- Difficulty organising care plan meetings or reviews
- Little engagement or involvement of the partner
- No *one* professional taking responsibility for co-ordinating care

For **midwives**, delivering care to this client group can be very time consuming. Committed midwives can often spend considerable time co-ordinating care, liaising with other professionals, organising antenatal and postnatal care planning meetings, organising the additional antenatal care requirements that these women often need, and visiting in excess of 10 days postpartum. There should be an exit strategy for visiting midwives which includes a health visitor.

In addition to the organisational and service delivery difficulties there are a number of other reasons why the care of pregnant women with drug and/or alcohol related problems has been difficult for health and social care providers.

Ideology

The prevailing societal view of women with substance misuse problems is a negative one. Drug and alcohol dependent women have been characterised as irresponsible, inadequate, deviant, immoral and unfit for motherhood. Research shows that women who are drug or alcohol dependent get significantly more social disapproval than men.[4] In pregnancy, this view is heightened as the welfare of the unborn child is emphasised and assumptions are made about the harmful consequences of the mother's drug/alcohol use and her ability to be a 'good mother' and care adequately for her child.[5] This gender bias has led to punitive responses, unacceptable levels of surveillance and restricted options for treatment

4. *Klee, Jackson and Lewis 2002*
5. *Macrory and Crosby 1995*

and care.[6] Negative societal views and professional attitudes coupled with discriminatory practice have deterred women from seaking help. They may appear to neglect their condition and that of their babies but in reality it may be the service's attitudes and approach that have excluded them from care.[7]

Research evidence

Lack of good data and research evidence on the effects of illicit drug use on the foetus and baby has led to some confusion and exaggeration of risk. Providing balanced and factual information to women so that they can make informed choices in pregnancy has proved difficult and women continue to receive inconsistent and contradictory advice.

Women's fears

Not surprisingly, pregnant women who have substance misuse problems frequently report a number of concerns including:

- Fear of being automatically referred to social work
- Fear that her baby will be taken into care
- Fear and confusion over whether her drug use will cause foetal damage
- Fear that she will be blamed if anything goes wrong with her pregnancy
- Fear of being thought of as an uncaring or 'unfit' mother if she doesn't manage to come off or reduce her drug use
- Feeling guilty and 'to blame' for her baby experiencing withdrawal symptoms

Poor social circumstances

Drug and alcohol related problems are commonly associated with socio-economic deprivation and poor social circumstances. These include:

- Poor support from family and friends
- Poor support from a substance-misusing partner
- Drug related criminal activity and legal problems (e.g. outstanding charges, impending court cases, community service order, probation, prison history, drug treatment and testing orders)
- Current or past history of sexual abuse
- Violence (e.g. substance misuse-related or domestic abuse)

6. Klee, Jackson & Lewis 2002
7. Morrison 1999

- Financial problems (including debts, fines and problems with welfare benefits)
- Housing problems (including homelessness, insecure or unsuitable housing)

Maternal health problems

Injecting drug use and *harmful levels of drinking* are associated with poor maternal health. This may include:
- Malnutrition and anaemia
- Respiratory problems
- Poor dental hygiene
- Blood-borne virus infections (HIV, hepatitis B, hepatitis C)
- Complications from injecting (such as abscesses, endocarditis, septicaemia etc)
- Liver disease
- Accidental injury
- Overdose and maternal death
- Mental health problems (such as anxiety, depression, self harm, psychosis)

Chaotic lifestyle

Drug and alcohol related problems are commonly associated with a *chaotic lifestyle* and may result in the woman receiving *poor maternity care.* For example:
- Late pregnancy booking
- Poor attendance for antenatal care
- Not registering with a general practitioner
- Poor attendance for parenthood education
- Late presentation during labour
- Early discharge home after delivery

Obstetric and paediatric problems

Drug use (including alcohol and tobacco) impacts on *obstetric* and *paediatric* morbidity and mortality. Increased rates of *low birth weight, pre-term delivery, Sudden Infant Death Syndrome* (SIDS or 'cot death') and *Neonatal Abstinence Syndrome* (NAS) in babies are the most commonly reported problems. The effects of specific substances on the developing foetus and baby are outlined later in the book (see page 28).

It is well established that many obstetric problems associated with substance misuse *are also* associated with social deprivation, poor antenatal care, poor maternal health and nutrition.[8] A number of case controlled studies have found comparable outcomes in women (who are matched by age, parity, social deprivation category etc) who *do not* have substance misuse problems.[9] Social factors, as well as the quality of health and social care provision, significantly influence the health and well being of both mother and baby.

8. *Mounteney 1999*
9. *Siney 1999*

Framework for care

A number of recent governmental publications have provided a broad set of principles and guidelines on good practice for working with pregnant women and families affected by drug and alcohol related problems. These include:

- *Drug Misuse and Dependence – Guidelines on Clinical Management*, Annex 5: *Pregnancy and Neonatal Care*, Department of Health (1999)
- *A Framework for Maternity Services in Scotland*, Scottish Executive (2001)
- *Integrated Care for Drug Users*, Effective Interventions Unit (2002)
- *Plan for Action on Alcohol Problems*, Scottish Executive (2002)
- *Getting Our Priorities Right*, Scottish Executive (2003)
- *Hidden Harm: responding to the needs of children of problem drug users*, the Advisory Council on the Misuse of Drugs report (2003)
- *Why Mothers Die 2000–2002*, 6th report (2004), Confidential Enquiry into Maternal and Child Health (CEMACH)
- Maternity Services in *The National Service Framework for Children, Young People and Maternity Services*, Department of Health (2004).

Philosophy of approach

The philosophy of approach outlined here reflects the central themes from these policy documents as well as recommendations from leading experts in the field.

Overall, the approach to care needs to be:

- women and family centred
- non-judgemental
- pragmatic, with an emphasis on harm reduction
- holistic
- provided by a multi-disciplinary and multi-agency team

Women and family centred approach

Pregnancy and the transition into parenthood is a significant life event. For women who have problems related to alcohol and drug misuse it offers opportunities as well as risks. These women have the *same hopes and aspirations* for family life and the same anxieties about pregnancy, childbirth and motherhood as other women.[10]

For service providers, the challenge is to offer the right kind of support that will allow them to *minimise the risks* as much as possible and to *make the most of*

---

10. Ford and Hepburn 1997

available opportunities. This means that treatment and care needs to be *women* and *family centred.*

The important role of partners needs to be recognised, and professionals need to ensure that, where appropriate, they are encouraged and supported to take a full and active role in pregnancy, childbirth and postnatal care. Women and their partners need to be able to make fully informed choices about their care. They need timely, relevant and *easily accessible* information to help them make the choices they face. They also need *prompt access* to any treatment and care that they might need.

Maternity care should be tailored to the needs of the individual woman and her family, focusing on the safety of mother and baby. It should take into account:
- the needs and wishes of the woman and her family
- her right to privacy and dignity throughout her pregnancy
- her cultural values, beliefs, attitudes, and chosen lifestyle

A *family centred approach* will create an atmosphere of normalisation and partnership that will engage the woman and her partner and foster the best possible outcome for mother and baby.

Non-judgemental approach

Service providers need to adopt a truly professional approach that is not led by views which are distorted by prejudice or limited by conventional stereotypes.[11] Professionals need to continually examine their approach to care so that they can account for their practice in terms of what is in the best interests of the woman and her baby and what is in accordance with the *best available evidence* and *best practice.*

Establishing early contact with pregnant women who have substance misuse problems and retaining them in treatment and care is vital.

This can best be achieved by creating a *non-judgemental environment.* Providing care with compassion, reassurance and encouragement will facilitate good contact. A non-judgemental approach is also a pre-requisite for obtaining the necessary details of the woman's substance misuse and social circumstances.

The woman needs to feel *supported* throughout her pregnancy and beyond. This

---

11. *Klee, Jackson and Lewis 2002*

means that professionals need to create a *positive pregnancy experience* for the woman, irrespective of risk and despite any difficulties that she may have.

Harm reduction approach

Substance misuse in pregnancy is associated with increased risks. Pregnancy therefore provides an excellent opportunity for professionals to provide education and care within a *harm reduction framework*.[12] Harm reduction is a pragmatic approach to care which aims to reduce the harm to individuals and society whether or not it is possible to reduce the substance use *per se.* It is essentially a *public health policy* designed to minimise risk. It is a *reality-based* approach that focuses on what *could* be done rather than what *should* be done. A harm reduction approach includes providing the means, information and education to enable people to make informed choices about their lifestyle.

Treatment and care goals must be realistic and tailored to the needs of the individual woman. Pressurising pregnant women into reducing or coming off drugs may lead to more harm than good. A flexible service that is able to take account of the wishes of the woman and support her to make her own decisions and be guided by what she feels she can achieve, will be most successful.[13]

It is important to remember that a harm reduction approach *includes abstinence.* Abstinence can be helpfully thought of as the 'final goal' of harm reduction and one which many people with substance misuse problems may wish to achieve. Drug and alcohol *dependency* however, is considered a chronic relapsing condition. People may use drugs and alcohol in potentially harmful ways for *many* years before achieving abstinence.

Long-term support to help people *minimise the harm* associated with substance misuse is normally required and may include such interventions as: substitute prescribing; needle exchange; and safer drug use/sensible drinking advice and support.

Holistic approach

Pregnant women with substance misuse problems often present with a *multiplicity* of needs and their substance misuse is just one aspect of their lives. A *holistic*

12. *Johnstone 1998*
13. *McIntosh 2001*

approach to care, from preconception to parenthood, needs to be offered. A holistic assessment should aim to identify their physical, psychological and social needs. It encompasses the *context* and *causes* of their problems and addresses the needs of other family members. A holistic package of care recognises that a woman's needs are inter-related and aims to provide a service that can address not just one aspect of her care, but all her needs and current strengths.

Multi-disciplinary and multi-agency approach

Pregnant women, whose drug or alcohol use is likely to impact on the outcome of their pregnancy, will need a comprehensive service provided by a multi-professional team. This service should provide consistent advice and support and continuity of care and aim to ensure safety for both mother and baby.

Many women will benefit from receiving care from a range of health and social care providers. This *multi-agency approach* to care needs to be well co-ordinated and integrated. Good communication between professionals is central to the provision of good quality care. Integrated care is where everyone involved in the provision of care has a shared philosophy of approach, knows what each other is doing and saying, and also knows what the woman herself wants.

A clear understanding of *professional roles and responsibilities* is needed to maximise the quality of care. Collaborative working should minimise the opportunities for contradictory or opinion-based advice and practice. Professionals delivering care need to have the *knowledge and skills* necessary for the type and level of service they provide. They should be aware of the expertise of other professionals and be prepared to draw upon that expertise where needed.

Pregnant women with substance misuse problems should receive the same quality of care, respect and dignity as any other pregnant woman throughout their pregnancy. The philosophy of approach outlined above and the guidelines on good practice that follow should ensure that this should be achieved.

Guidelines on good practice

This section of the book outlines *guidelines on good practice* for working with pregnant women who have substance misuse problems.

The care process

It is important that all professionals involved with substance-misusing women follow a clear 'pathway of care', from pre-conception through to parenthood. A template model 'care pathway' is included as an example in appendix 2.

The care process involves *assessment*, planning care and agreeing an individual *care plan*, *implementing* care, and *reviewing* care. These key tasks in the care process are outlined below, along with a *checklist* of topics that are relevant to each stage of the process, many of which are covered in the course of routine health care as well as drug and alcohol treatment and social care service provision.

Assessment

Assessment should be holistic and continuous throughout pregnancy. It should take into account the woman's physical and psychological health needs, her social circumstances, her partner's drug and alcohol use, an assessment of risk as well as her own drug use (including alcohol and tobacco). *It may involve a number of different professionals contributing to the assessment process over time*, including the General Practitioner, midwifery, obstetric and paediatric staff, the Health Visitor, Drug and Alcohol Worker and Social Worker.

An assessment of **physical health needs** should include such topics a
- Past obstetric/gynaecological history
- General health status
- Nutrition (e.g. diet, weight, anaemia)
- Dental health
- Exposure to infections (e.g. blood-borne viruses, sexually transmitted infections)
- Complications from injecting (including venous access and DVT)
- Accidents or injuries
- Difficulty getting registered with GP

An assessment of **psychological needs** should include such topics as:
- Was the baby planned?
- Was abortion considered?

- Worries or concerns about pregnancy (e.g. fear baby will be taken into care, fear of damage to the foetus)
- Current or past anxiety related problems
- Current low mood or history of depression/self harm
- History of eating disorder (e.g. anorexia or bulimia)
- Low self esteem or self worth
- History of physical, emotional or sexual abuse
- Bereavement issues
- Woman's perception of her own circumstances, needs and coping ability

An assessment of **social needs** should include:
- Housing situation (e.g. homelessness, insecure or unsuitable accommodation)
- Financial situation (e.g. debts, rent arrears, unpaid bills or fines)
- Legal situation (e.g. current charges, impending court cases, community service or probation orders, drug treatment and testing orders)
- Employment or training and education issues
- Care of any existing children
- Parenting skills
- Relationships with partner, family, friends
- Available social support network
- Contact with other health and social care workers

An **assessment of drug use** should include the following:
- Smoking
- Alcohol use
- Illicit (street) drug use
- Injecting drug use
- Prescribed drug use
- Use of 'over the counter' medications
- Current contact with specialist drug/alcohol services
- Current treatment and care goals
- Previous contact with drug/alcohol services

An assessment of the **partner's drug use** should include:
- Partner's current use of tobacco, alcohol and drugs
- Level of stability if drug dependent
- Is partner currently injecting drugs?
- Blood-borne virus (HIV, HCV, HBV) status?
- Partner's current contact with health and social care agencies

A **risk assessment** should include:
- Obstetric/gynaecological problems
- Current maternal health problems
- Domestic abuse
- Previous history of child care problems
- Impact of substance misuse on lifestyle
- Impact of drug culture environment
- Social isolation/unsupported pregnancy
- Parenting history of woman and partner
- Current engagement in prostitution

Care planning

Care should be planned in **partnership** with the woman and, where appropriate, her partner. Care planning involves developing a *'package of care'* that meets the woman's needs and takes account of her views and wishes. It includes what treatment and care will be provided, and by whom, as well as the desired outcomes. Care plans need to be *realistic* and *achievable* and they should include a *date for* review.[14] This, ideally, should be arranged for between 28–32 weeks gestation.

A **care plan** would include some or all of the following:
- Antenatal care including screening tests, scans, monitoring of foetal growth
- Treatment and care of substance misuse (realistic harm reduction goals and strategies)
- Plan to address any social needs
- Plan to meet and involve the partner in care (where appropriate)
- Preparation for parenthood (including parent education classes)
- Preparation for childbirth (labour and delivery)
- Preparation for Neonatal Abstinence Syndrome (if drug dependent)
- Preparation for infant feeding (support and encouragement to breastfeed)
- Plan for postnatal care (including preparations for infant and social support)
- Plan to address any risks or concerns associated with parenting skills or child care
- Plan to involve other professionals and referral to other agencies
- Plan for multi-disciplinary/multi-agency meeting/child protection case conference

14. *Whittaker and McLeod 1998*

Reviewing the care plan

The *care plan* and *progress of care* need to be reviewed at *regular intervals* throughout the pregnancy (for example at each antenatal appointment).

Women with identified risks or multiple social needs may benefit from attending an organised 'care plan review' meeting. All parties involved in the delivery of care should be encouraged to attend review meetings or submit a brief report. If the care plan review meeting takes place around 28 weeks gestation then there will be enough time for services to be put in place in time for the arrival of the baby.

The **review process** should include a discussion on the following topics:
- Attendance for antenatal care?
- Foetal health and development?
- Maternal health? (including mental health)
- Current smoking/alcohol/drug use?
- Attendance for other health care appointments? (e.g. GP, Health Visitor or Community Mental Health Nurse)
- Attendance at specialist drug/alcohol service?
- Attendance for social care appointments? (e.g. social work, voluntary sector agencies)
- Involvement and support of partner?
- Stability of lifestyle?
- Improvement in social circumstances?
- Current or potential risks?
- Future needs to address?
- Future goals to work towards?

Care management

Some women with substance misuse problems and their families will have *complex* health and social care needs and will require a *care management* approach and a *comprehensive package of care* during pregnancy and well into the postnatal period. In these cases, one professional needs to be identified as the *care co-ordinator* to take responsibility for managing the care process. The role of this 'lead professional' is to ensure that the care process is fully documented, implemented and reviewed. This requires good liaison, communication and organisational skills to ensure a continuum of care is delivered in accordance with the agreed care plan for the family.

Consent to share information with other professionals

All professionals working with pregnant women who have substance misuse problems need to work *collaboratively* with other professionals and agencies in order to provide good quality care. It is important to discuss 'joint working' with the woman at an *early stage* so that **informed consent** can be obtained to allow information sharing. Most women are happy to agree to this once the benefits of inter-agency collaboration are explained. Information regarding her assessment, care plan and progress can then be exchanged between professionals.

Although the woman may consent to 'joint working' she may still need reassurance about her right to privacy and should be given guidance on the Data Protection Act (1998) and the terms of professional **confidentiality**. This will include advice about circumstances whereby confidentiality may be breached e.g. for child protection, mental health or legal reasons. A *proforma* **consent form** is included as an example in appendix 3. The consent form can be photocopied and sent to all professionals involved in the woman's care (i.e. the Midwife, GP, Health Visitor, Drug/Alcohol worker, Social Worker etc).

Information and guidelines on drug use

Ideally, all professionals who provide care to pregnant women with substance misuse problems should be able to:

- Provide information on the risks associated with drug use in pregnancy
- Assess drug and alcohol related problems in pregnancy
- Provide advice about how to manage drug use in pregnancy
- Discuss substance misuse treatment and care options for pregnancy

If professionals cannot provide the above then they should ensure that they refer women to services that can.

Trends in substance use (illicit and prescribed)

This section of the book includes basic information on commonly used drugs.

Commonly used drugs include:

- **cannabis** (hash and marijuana)
- **stimulants** (such as amphetamine, cocaine, ecstasy)
- **hallucinogens** (e.g. LSD and magic mushrooms)
- **opioids** (e.g. heroin, methadone, dihydrocodeine, buprenorphine)
- **benzodiazepines** (e.g. diazepam and temazepam)
- **volatile substances** (e.g. gas and glue)
- **other drugs** (such as cyclizine, ketamine, gammahydroxybutrate or 'GHB', 'poppers', steroids, anti-depressants).

Most women who use drugs do not inject them. Oral 'polydrug' use is more common. Cannabis is the most widely used illicit drug and is normally mixed with tobacco and smoked in a 'joint' or 'spliff'. Central nervous system (CNS) **stimulant** drugs, such as amphetamine, ecstasy and cocaine, are commonly used for recreational purposes and are popular in the dance club social scene. **Anti-depressants** (mostly SSRIs) are also in widespread use. They are prescribed for the treatment of depression and anxiety related problems and can interact with other CNS depressant drugs and CNS stimulant drugs.

Effects of commonly used drugs

Benzodiazepine drugs, such as diazepam (Valium) and temazepam, are commonly called minor tranquillisers or sleeping tablets (hypnotics) and are CNS depressant drugs. They are easily available on the black market and are in widespread use. People can become dependent on benzodiazepines in a very short period of time if they are used continuously. Sudden withdrawal from benzodiazepines can result in severe anxiety symptoms, hallucinations and seizures (similar to alcohol dependency withdrawal symptoms). Panic attacks caused by benzodiazepines may be a reason for not attending ante-natal appointments.

Opioid drugs are CNS depressant drugs that have an analgesic (pain killer) effect. They include:

- opiates: derived from the opium poppy e.g. morphine and codeine, and their
- synthetic analogues, e.g. methadone (meth), diamorphine (heroin), dihydrocodeine (DF118 or 'difs'), dipipanone (Diconal), pethidine.

Opioids produce a range of physical effects apart from analgesia. They depress nervous system activity, including reflex functions such as coughing, respiration and heart rate. They also depress bowel activity, resulting in constipation. At higher doses sedation results and the user becomes drowsy and contented. Excessive doses produce stupor and coma. Tolerance and physical dependence develops with regular continued use. The physiological effects of long-term opiate use are rarely serious in themselves. They include respiratory complaints, constipation and menstrual irregularity.

Opioid intoxication An intoxicated person may be unresponsive, have pinpoint pupils, respiratory depression (shallow and infrequent breathing), a weak and rapid pulse, and they may appear pale and have cold extremities.

Opioid overdose is life threatening. Immediate medical attention and treatment is required (normally *naloxone* is administered to reverse the effects of overdose). A person who has taken an overdose will have blue lips and cold skin, will lose consciousness and not respond to stimuli, develop respiratory failure and may die (sometimes through asphyxia after vomiting).

Opioid withdrawal in adults Abrupt withdrawal is rarely life-threatening and is considered less dangerous than withdrawal from alcohol or benzodiazepines. Withdrawal symptoms develop in dependent opiate users normally 24–72 hours after their last dose. Symptoms can include: nausea, vomiting, diarrhoea, insomnia, muscle cramps, goose flesh, cold and clammy skin, dilated pupils, runny nose and eyes, abdominal pains, sweating, restlessness, irritability, as well as intense craving for the drug. Physical symptoms normally subside without treatment within 7 days.

Injecting drug use

Although most women drug users report taking drugs by oral administration (swallowing, snorting or smoking), *injecting drug use* is on the increase. Drugs that can be easily prepared for injection include:

- diamorphine (heroin)
- buprenorphine (Temgesic, Subutex)
- dipipanone (Diconal)
- cyclizine (Valoid)
- amphetamines (speed)
- cocaine

Injecting drug use and sharing needles and syringes and other injecting paraphernalia (e.g. spoons, filters, water etc) remains a major public health concern. Messages about the risks associated with *sharing* injecting paraphernalia need to be continually emphasised by professionals as many young drug users do not perceive themselves to be at risk of blood-borne viruses (HIV, hepatitis C and hepatitis B). It is now standard practice that all pregnant women are offered HIV and hepatitis B testing as part of ante-natal screening. While testing for hepatitis C is not routine, it is recommended for drug users.

Drugs and their effects on the developing baby

All women should be given information on the effects of smoking, alcohol use and drug use in pregnancy. Ideally, information should be given well before *conception* so that the woman has an opportunity to modify her drug use *before* she becomes pregnant.

The general answer to a question like 'I took some x before I found out I was pregnant. Is it likely to harm the baby?' is almost certainly 'no'. However, outcomes depend on the drug used, the amount taken, over what time period, how it was taken, at what stage in pregnancy, and many other factors such as diet and social circumstances. One unfortunate aspect of over-emphasising the likelihood of adverse effects is that it may persuade some concerned women to inappropriately consider termination.[15] Others may suddenly stop their dependent drug use (which could be dangerous to the foetus) or avoid engaging with professionals because of exaggerated concerns.

Drug use is associated with increased rates of obstetric and paediatric mortality and morbidity and can affect pregnancy in a number of ways. During the first trimester, when foetal organs are actually forming, *teratogenic* (malformation) effects are the main concern. This is a time when the woman may not even know she is pregnant. During the second and third trimester the main concern is about *growth and functional* development.[16] Impaired placental function and foetal growth can result in a *low birth weight* baby. Chaotic drug use can increase the risk of *pre-term labour* and result in early delivery. The risk of *Sudden Infant Death Syndrome (SIDS)* is increased and *Neonatal Abstinence Syndrome* is common in the babies of women who are dependent on certain drugs.

Many women with alcohol/drug related problems feel *worried* and *guilty* about the effects of their drug use on the baby and may *appear* reluctant to discuss these issues as a result.[17] Professionals need to give parents license to voice concerns, fears and questions that they are reluctant to bring up spontaneously.

Very often parents will be relieved when a professional *raises the subject* and *encourages* them to share their concerns. Allowing them to voice anxieties about poor outcome and their ambivalence about their current situation, including their substance use, treatment and so on can be therapeutic. Parents often complain that they are not 'told enough' and professionals comment that parents are 'ill prepared' or 'ill informed'.

15. *Mounteney 1999*
16. *Siney 1999*
17. *Klee, Jackson and Lewis 2002*

Evidence base

It has been difficult to establish clear and reliable information about the effects of specific drugs on the developing foetus and baby. Much of the research is *methodologically flawed* and findings are inconsistent and contradictory. This is because well-controlled studies are difficult to conduct and *pregnancy outcome is multifactorial*. It is the result of an interplay of genetic factors, physical and psychological health, nutrition, health and social care, social deprivation and other environmental influences as well as the effects of tobacco, alcohol and drug use. These *confounding factors* have made it difficult to establish *cause-and-effect* relationships. This is particularly true when relating specific intrauterine foetal drug exposure to long-term behavioural effects as the child grows up.[18]

Drug and alcohol related problems are associated with poverty, unemployment, chaotic lifestyle, violence, poor physical and psychological health and poor uptake of health and social care. These other factors may therefore account for many of the findings reported in the research literature. There is also a moral dimension to what purports to be objective scientific evidence.[19] Reports of adverse effects are more likely to be published than research reporting no adverse effects, irrespective of the scientific validity of the research.[20] The following information on *specific* drug effects should be read with these *limitations* in mind.

Effects of tobacco

The significant risks associated with maternal use of tobacco are particularly well established. There are many harmful substances contained in cigarettes. Nicotine, carbon monoxide and cyanide are thought to have the greatest adverse effects, reducing blood flow and oxygen to the foetus.

Women who smoke during their pregnancy are three times more likely to have a *low birthweight* baby and stillbirths or early neonatal deaths are 30 per cent higher among women who smoke. Smoking tobacco causes a reduction in birth weight *greater* than that from heroin and is a major risk factor in *Sudden Infant Death Syndrome* (SIDS).[21]

18. Johnstone 1998
19. Mounteney 1999
20. Koren et al 1982
21. www.dh.gov.uk/PublicationsAndStatistics see also www.sids.org.uk/fsid

Although there is no convincing evidence that smoking cigarettes causes congenital birth defects, many other pregnancy complications are associated with smoking.[22] These include:

- miscarriage
- pre-term (premature) delivery
- stillbirth
- intrauterine growth restriction (IUGR) or 'small for dates'
- low birth weight
- placental abruption
- reduction in breast milk production
- Sudden Infant Death Syndrome (SIDS or 'cot death').

Babies born to heavy smokers may also exhibit minor signs of withdrawal, including 'jitteriness' in the perinatal period. Children of smokers also suffer more respiratory infections in childhood and adolescence.

Effects of alcohol

Alcohol use during pregnancy may potentially affect foetal brain development at any gestation. At all points along the continuum from occasional light drinking to regular heavy drinking there is conflicting evidence as to the possibility of damaging effects on the foetus.[23]

It is important to remember that a 'safe' level of alcohol use in pregnancy has not been established.

Low levels (<7 units per week) of alcohol use during pregnancy appear to cause little harm for the baby, although in the first trimester it has been associated with an increased risk of *miscarriage.*[24]

Maternal consumption of 15 units or more per week has been associated with a reduction in *birth weight.*

Consumption of 20 units or more per week has been associated with *intellectual impairment* in children.

Very heavy drinking in pregnancy (including heavy 'binge' drinking) results in a small number of babies being born with *Foetal Alcohol Syndrome* (FAS).

22. Johnstone 1998
23. Mounteney 1999
24. Taylor 2003

Foetal Alcohol Syndrome is characterised by:

- Foetal *growth restriction* (with subsequent *low birth weight*, reduced head circumference and brain size)
- *Central nervous system problems*, including cognitive dysfunction (learning difficulties) and neurological abnormalities
- A cluster of characteristic *facial abnormalities* e.g. short palpebral fissures (eye openings), thin upper lip, flattened midface and indistinct philtrum
- *Failure to thrive* (the child remains below the 10th centile)

Studies that report alcohol consumption related to FAS have found high levels of drinking (>42 units per week). *Patterns of consumption* also seem to be important. Frequent high dose ('binge') drinking, to the point of intoxication, is thought to be a greater risk to the foetus than steady moderate drinking. Many other *confounding factors* however, may be important. These include general physical health, nutrition, age, parity, smoking and other drug use as well as social deprivation.[25]

A wide range of other alcohol-related birth defects (ARBD) appear to occur with heavy drinking. These *foetal alcohol effects* include more subtle problems identified on behavioural, cognitive, psychological and educational tests.

Effects of drugs (illicit and prescribed)

As stated earlier, studies examining the effects of drugs in pregnancy are fraught with methodological difficulties and multiple confounding variables producing inconsistent and contradictory findings.

Drug effects on the foetus are *broadly similar* and largely *non-specific*. Intrauterine growth restriction (IUGR) and pre-term deliveries contribute to increased rates of low birth weight and increased perinatal mortality rate. These outcomes are *multi-factorial* and are also associated with socio-economic deprivation, poor maternal health and smoking.[26]

Cannabis

Despite its widespread use, information on the effects of cannabis in pregnancy is generally poor. A review of cannabis by the World Health Organisation (1997)

---

25. *Plant 1997, Abel 1998*
26. *Department of Health 1999*

concluded that there was no good evidence that cannabis itself has a direct effect on pregnancy or the developing baby. Cannabis however, is normally mixed together with tobacco and smoked in a 'joint'. Tobacco causes a reduction in birth weight, increased risk of sudden infant death syndrome (SIDS or 'cot death') and many other pregnancy complications (see page 29). Excessive use of cannabis may be symptomatic of other unresolved issues. Asking about cannabis use may reveal use of other, more dangerous drugs like crack.

Benzodiazepines (e.g. diazepam and temazepam)

There is no conclusive evidence that benzodiazepine use by the mother causes adverse effects on the developing foetus. Most studies however, have studied low dose use. There have been some reports of facial abnormalities (i.e. cleft lip and palate) following prolonged high dose benzodiazepine use in early pregnancy but these findings have not been reliably reproduced.[27]

Benzodiazepines are associated with *withdrawal symptoms* in the newborn baby that can be severe and prolonged (see section on NAS, page 35). Because of concerns about the possible increased risk of cleft palate, reduced growth and brain development and long-term outcomes for the baby, dependent women are normally advised to *gradually reduce* their benzodiazepine use during pregnancy.

Opioids (e.g. heroin and methadone)

Evidence on the effects of opioids is fairly limited, particularly on the long-term effects on the child. Opioids are associated with an increased risk of:

- *low birth weight*
- intrauterine growth restriction (IUGR) or *'small for dates'*
- *pre-term delivery* (associated with foetal withdrawal in-utero, poor diet and maternal health)
- *Sudden Infant Death Syndrome* (SIDS or 'cot death').

There is no convincing evidence that opioids cause any significant or permanent neurological damage or increased risk of congenital abnormalities.[28]

Abrupt withdrawal of opiates (i.e. 'cold turkey') has been associated with *miscarriage* in the first trimester and *stillbirth* and *pre-term labour* in the third

27. *Johnstone 1998*
28. *Ibid.*

trimester. Sudden opiate withdrawal is therefore considered potentially dangerous to the foetus, although the risks of withdrawal have probably been exaggerated in the past and can be minimised by appropriate drug therapy for the mother.[29] Most studies that report these findings relate to women with a history of *injecting* opiate use (primarily heroin) and chaotic *illicit* drug use.

Neonatal Abstinence Syndrome (NAS or 'neonatal withdrawal') is well documented in babies born to opiate dependent women and is the most commonly reported effect of opiate use in pregnancy.

Cocaine and Crack

Cocaine is a powerful vasoconstrictor (restricting blood flow and oxygen to the foetus) and this effect is reported to increase the risk of:

- *placental abruption* (placental separation with haemorrhage and foetal hypoxia)
- *intrauterine growth restriction* (including reduced brain growth)
- underdevelopment of organs and/or limbs
- *foetal death in-utero* (miscarriage and stillbirth)
- *low birth weight* babies
- *pre-term* (premature) delivery

Adverse effects have been largely reported in heavy crack/cocaine users, rather than with 'recreational' or occasional users. Cocaine 'binges' can potentially cause foetal brain infarcts due to sudden reduced blood flow.[30] **Mothers-to-be should be advised not to use cocaine or crack in pregnancy if they possibly can.**

High dose cocaine use in the mother can result in the newborn showing *signs of intoxication* at birth that include: 'jitteriness', irritability, hypertonia, poor feeding and an abnormal sleep pattern.

Dependent crack/cocaine users should be managed by the consultant obstetrician and referred to a specialist drug agency for help. A course of acupuncture may help with cocaine cravings.

29. Johnstone 1998
30. Ford and Hepburn 1997

Amphetamines (e.g. 'speed' or 'whizz')

There is no conclusive evidence that amphetamine use directly affects pregnancy outcomes. However, amphetamine sulphate is a powerful CNS stimulant and heavy users tend to have poor health (due to poor nutrition, weight loss, anaemia and mental health problems). Like cocaine, amphetamines cause vasoconstriction and hypertension, which may result in foetal hypoxia.

Withdrawal symptoms in the newborn baby have not been reliably reported with amphetamine use. As with other drugs, in the absence of good data, advice should be to avoid or at least reduce intake during pregnancy.[31]

Ecstasy ('E')

There is no conclusive evidence that ecstasy use directly affects pregnancy outcomes, however information in the literature is very scarce. Heavy users of ecstasy may have poor physical and mental health (e.g. depression) and this may affect outcome. Ecstasy use by the mother does not appear to cause withdrawal symptoms in the newborn baby.

Hallucinogens
(e.g. LSD – lysergic acid diethylamide or 'acid' – and 'Magic Mushrooms')

There is little evidence regarding the effects of hallucinogens in pregnancy. There is no evidence of congenital malformations and no conclusive evidence of other increased risks in pregnancy.

Solvents and volatile substances (e.g. 'glue' and butane gas)

There is little evidence regarding the effects of solvent and volatile substance use in pregnancy. However, inhaled solvents may reduce oxygen supply to the foetus and Neonatal Abstinence Syndrome has been reported in heavy users. Women who continue to use volatile substances in pregnancy run the risk of sudden death.[32]

31. *Johnstone 1998*
32. *Johnstone 1998*

Neonatal Abstinence Syndrome (NAS)

A group of drug withdrawal symptoms referred to as *Neonatal Abstinence Syndrome* (NAS) can occur in infants born to mothers dependent on certain drugs. NAS occurs because, at birth, the infant is cut off from the maternal drug supply to which it has been exposed *in utero*. NAS is the most commonly reported adverse effect of dependent drug use in pregnancy.

The classes of drugs that are known to cause NAS include the opioids, benzodiazepines, alcohol, and barbiturates. Classical symptoms of NAS have not been consistently reported with solvents, hallucinogens, cannabis and most stimulants. NAS symptoms are generally non-specific to the class of drug and differ from drug withdrawal symptoms seen in adults.

NAS is well described in babies born to *opiate dependent women*. The majority of infants born to dependent mothers (60–90 per cent) will show varying symptoms of NAS.

Signs and symptoms of NAS

NAS is characterised by central nervous system irritability, gastro-intestinal dysfunction and autonomic hyperactivity.

The following signs and symptoms have been reported in babies born to opiate and benzodiazepine dependent women (including polydrug users) and describe the more *severe* range of symptoms that a baby may display:

- irritability (marked tremor, easily startled, increased reflexes and excessive crying)
- hyperactivity (excessive body movements, face scratching)
- hypertonicity (increased muscle tone and rigidity)
- a fairly continuous high-pitched cry
- inability to settle or sleep after feeds
- excessive sucking (including fist sucking)
- increased appetite
- poor feeding ability (hungry but difficulty in sucking, swallowing and successfully completing a feed)
- regurgitation and vomiting
- frequent loose stools or diarrhoea (which cause peri-anal excoriation)
- poor weight gain or weight loss
- repetitive sneezing, yawning, hiccoughs, nasal stuffiness
- tachypnoea (rapid shallow breathing)

- respiratory depression
- increased pulse and heart rate
- temperature instability, fever (>37.5 C), sweating and dehydration
- mottling (discolouration of skin)
- excoriation (skin abrasions) from excessive movement (usually seen around the buttocks, back of the head, shoulders, and heels)
- seizures (fits)

Seizures occur rarely (in approximately 5 per cent of infants) and may manifest up to 30 days after birth (mean age of onset is 10 days).

The onset, duration and severity of NAS symptoms vary greatly and depend on many factors, including the:
- type of drugs used
- duration of mother's dependency
- timing and amount of the mother's last dose
- metabolism and elimination of the drug by the infant, as well as the
- gestational age of the infant

Data on possible dose related effects of methadone are inconclusive.[33] Some studies show no correlation between maternal methadone dose and the development or severity of NAS. Others have found a weak positive correlation. Little data exists on the dose related effects of maternal benzodiazepine use.

Symptoms normally present within the first 24–72 hours of birth (in approximately 75 per cent of cases). Methadone withdrawal in the neonate can present *later* than heroin withdrawal. Methadone withdrawal symptoms can also *last longer* and be *more severe.*[34]

The onset of benzodiazepine withdrawal in neonates can also be delayed (due to slow metabolism in the neonate) presenting at 5–10 days of age.[35]

Acute symptoms of NAS may persist for several weeks and irritability can last for some months (particularly from benzodiazepines). *Pharmacological* treatment is required for some infants with acute symptoms (approximately 25 per cent – 40 per cent). Most studies show that babies who require treatment develop symptoms within 72 hours of birth, including babies born to methadone dependent women.[36]

33. Johnstone 1998
34. Sparey and Wilkinshaw 1999
35. Coghlan et al 1999
36. Shaw and McIvor 1994

Withdrawal symptoms in **pre-term infants** tend to occur later than full-term infants and are generally milder and require less treatment.[37] This is thought to be due to a number of different factors, including: their reduced total drug exposure *in utero*, the developmental immaturity of their central nervous system, the different metabolism of pre-term infants, and reduced ability to communicate the distress of withdrawal.

Some babies may present with symptoms of NAS with *no reported history* of maternal drug use. If NAS is suspected then the neonatal paediatrician can confirm the diagnosis by toxicology and will discuss the results sensitively with the parents.

Assessment of NAS

Assessment of the infant is best done using a standardised tool or *formal assessment score chart* as this provides the *most* objective measure of symptoms and the best guide for making decisions about treatment and care.[38]

Assessment can be carried out in a number of ways including the use of either the *Lipsitz tool* or a modified version of the *Finnegan* chart (see an example of a parent friendly NAS score chart in appendix 9), where numerical values are allocated on the basis of the presence and severity of various symptoms. The main dimensions that are measured include *irritability* symptoms (high-pitched cry, sleep pattern, body movements etc) and *gastrointestinal* symptoms (feeding pattern, weight, skin excoriation etc).

A score is allocated to each symptom for each time period (e.g. 9am–1pm, 1pm–5pm, etc). Total scores for each time period are then calculated and trends in the severity of the baby's condition are monitored. Any drug treatment administered is also recorded on the chart. This allows the medical staff to monitor the effectiveness of the drug treatment and to titrate the dose according to the infant's presenting symptoms, weaning the baby off gradually.

Applying the NAS score chart to *pre-term* infants can cause difficulties as symptoms such as high pitched cry, poor feeding and tachypnoea could be *over scored*, whilst other symptoms such as sleep pattern, muscle tone and fever could be *underscored*. Pre-term infants are cared for in hospital so staff should seek

37. Doberczak et al 1991
38. Shaw 1999

advice from the neonatal paediatrician. Many services are moving to amore holistic view of the baby's behaviour rather than simply relying on numerical values which can be interpreted subjectively.

All maternity staff should make themselves familiar with the current NAS score chart in use and be able to explain its use to parents.

Preparing parents for NAS

It is important to prepare parents for the possibility that their baby might develop NAS (even if they are dependent on very low doses of medication) and to communicate this information to them sensitively, using a non-judgemental approach.

Parents who have an infant with NAS experience the same range of emotions as any other parent of a newborn baby who is poorly. Anxiety, helplessness, fear and grief are commonly reported feelings. In addition they often feel guilty and 'to blame' for their baby's condition and will require considerable support, reassurance and encouragement. Caring for a baby with NAS can be very stressful and parents will require a lot of patience. Involving the parents in all the decisions and choices about their infants care and keeping them fully informed of the baby's progress is important.

Ideally, parents will have been given clear and accurate information about NAS in the *antenatal* period so that they are well prepared. At around 32 weeks, midwives should give all drug and alcohol dependent parents the information leaflet that come with this book *Caring for a baby with drug withdrawal symptoms* (see appendix 11). This leaflet outlines in 'user friendly' language, what parents can expect and how they can help. The woman and her partner should be advised to read the leaflet then discuss any questions or anxieties that they may have with the midwife. NAS is not life threatening and parents should be given advice and support on how to manage an irritable baby.

Management of neonatal withdrawal symptoms

The focus of care should be to:
- foster the maternal/infant bond
- ensure the safe adaptation of the baby to extra-uterine life
- detect any evidence of NAS symptoms and to offer appropriate treatment and care

Unnecessarily prolonged hospitalisation or placement away from the parents should be avoided if at all possible in an effort to keep mother and baby together, to enable effective breastfeeding and to promote good bonding.

All known drug dependent women should be asked to stay in hospital for a minimum of three days (72 hours) following delivery so that the neonate can be observed for signs and symptoms of NAS. Most babies with *mild to moderate* symptoms will be cared for in the *postnatal* ward. Staff in the postnatal ward should show parents how to use the NAS assessment score chart (see appendix 9) and encourage them to get involved in their baby's care from the very beginning. Parents should be advised to keep a close eye on their baby and report any concerns to staff.

Babies with mild symptoms *will not* require medical intervention and can be looked after using supportive *comfort* measures.

Supportive 'comfort' measures include:

- Provide a supportive environment (ensure minimal stimulation to the infant by decreasing stimuli in a quiet room with dim lighting, mild temperature, soft gentle music, no smoking near baby). If appropriate the mother should be offered a single room in hospital so that a suitable environment can be created for the baby.
- Recommend 'skin-to-skin' contact with mother to help regulate the baby's breathing and body temperature, relaxation and feeding.
- Swaddling of the baby will help with tremors, jerks and restlessness. When handling, wrap limbs (with arms and knees bent into a comfortable position) with a light soft flannel blanket, perhaps use a cotton baby sling.
- Ensure gentle handling of the baby, gentle wakening, gentle rocking, humming, perhaps try gentle baby massage and deep relaxation bath. Before disturbing the baby for changing, prepare everything that is needed.
- Provide a dummy or pacifier for non-nutritive sucking (except when breastfeeding). Cover the infant's hands with mittens to prevent trauma to fingers and fists.
- Ensure frequent changes of the baby's nappy. Use barrier creams to the skin around buttocks to prevent skin damage from frequent loose stools and excessive body movements.
- Feed the infant on demand, small frequent feeds are normally better and will reduce regurgitation and vomiting and prevent dehydration. Burp the infant

frequently as infants often swallow air due to their uncoordinated and poor sucking reflex.

- If the baby's sucking and swallowing reflex is poor then support the cheeks and lower jaw to enhance feeding.
- If the baby is being breast fed, feed in quiet, calm surroundings with minimal noise and disturbance and allow time for resting in-between sucking.
- Observe baby's temperature and remove blankets if fever is present. Clean skin and change clothes frequently if baby is sweating.

The use of supportive therapy has been shown to reduce the effects of withdrawal in neonates and should be implemented as soon as possible following birth. Parents should be encouraged to take a lead role in their infants' care and should be provided with this information so that they can care for their baby appropriately.

Please note: **naloxone** (an opiate antagonist) **should not be used** to reverse opioid induced respiratory depression in neonates as this will induce an abrupt opiate withdrawal crisis.

Care in the community

After 72 hours stay on the postnatal ward, babies with mild to moderate symptoms can be discharged home where they can be cared for by their *parents* with community midwifery and health visiting support. The midwife will offer advice and support on a daily basis and will arrange for readmission to hospital if the baby's symptoms worsen. As part of the infant's ongoing care, parents should be advised to continue using the NAS assessment score chart and supportive therapy measures until the baby's symptoms have resolved. Parents should be advised to *record* all feeds (amounts taken and times) so that the midwife and health visitor can monitor the baby's daily calorie intake. The community midwife and health visitor will also *weigh* the baby to ensure weight gain is satisfactory. Many areas now have specialist midwives situated in drug services who can offer additional support.

If the baby's symptoms get significantly worse at home (i.e. sleeps less than 1 hour/cries 1 hour after feeds/weight loss after day 7) then it is better to admit the baby to hospital *earlier* rather than later.

Care in hospital

Parents need to know that admission to their local neonatal or special care baby unit is necessary if their baby develops *severe* withdrawal symptoms.

Babies with severe symptoms often require 'tube' feeding, pharmacological (drug) treatment and 24-hour care and supervision from specialist paediatric medical and nursing staff.

The *aim* of treatment is to:
* reduce irritability and motor instability
* establish an appropriate *feed/sleep/wake* cycle
* maintain a normal body temperature, and
* ensure adequate weight gain.

Babies with severe symptoms may need to stay in the unit for about 10–14 days, but sometimes for much longer. Mothers should be encouraged to 'board' (rooms permitting) in the hospital whilst their baby is in the unit (particularly if they are breastfeeding) or at least have daily contact to continue the bonding process.

Pharmacological management is usually decided by the attending physician but normally includes the use of one or more of the following drugs: oral morphine, diazepam, clonazepam, clonidine, phenobarbitone, chlorpromazine or chloral hydrate. The best drug appears to be morphine if the main drug used by the mother has been an opioid. Where other drugs (e.g. benzodiazepines) have been used alone or in combination, drug therapy needs to be individually tailored towards a longer or biphasic pattern of withdrawal.[39]

Care is taken not to sedate the baby and to wean them off medication as soon as possible. Babies can be discharged home as soon as they are well enough to be cared for by their parents.

39. Shaw 1999

Management of substance use in pregnancy

Many women who are not truly dependent on alcohol or drugs will stop spontaneously as soon as they know they are pregnant. This applies to approximately 20 per cent of women who smoke and to many women who use cannabis and other drugs 'recreationally'. It also applies to some 'controlled' opiate and benzodiazepine users.[40] For most drug use (excluding opiates) the immediate goal would be one of abstinence, although in reality this may be difficult to achieve for many women. Much support and drug counselling may need to be offered to help the woman work towards this goal.

In addition, research shows that women who have substance misuse problems are more likely to have substance-misusing partners.[41] Substance-misusing sexual partners can exert a powerful influence over a woman's drug use. It is very important therefore, to include the woman's partner (where appropriate) in any treatment and care plan so that the most supportive environment can be created. Evidence suggests that women, who engage in treatment *with*, rather than without, their partner, have better outcomes.[42]

Smoking cessation

All women should be advised to stop smoking or given help to cut down, preferably *before* they conceive. General Practitioners can prescribe nicotine replacement therapy (NRT) and can refer to smoking cessation programmes. Bupropion (Zyban) can also help with nicotine cravings, however women who are pregnant or breastfeeding should not use bupropion.[43]

During pregnancy a pro-active approach to smoking cessation is required. Smoking cessation advice given in the antenatal period has been shown to be effective and can result in significant gains in birth weight.[44]

Many drug and alcohol dependent women however, may find it difficult to stop smoking. Pregnant women who are strongly nicotine dependent and unable to quit unaided, can be offered nicotine replacement therapy (NRT) following discussion with a health care professional. Although NRT is not licensed for use during pregnancy, a number of leading experts have put forward a rationale for treating pregnant smokers with NRT.[45] The use of NRT can benefit the mother and foetus if

40. Johnstone 1998
41. Effective Interventions Unit 2002
42. Ibid.
43. NICE 2002
44. Johnstone 1998
45. Wright and Walker 2001

it leads to cessation of smoking. Nicotine levels in the body whilst on NRT are typically lower than those present during heavy smoking and the many other toxins emitted by cigarette smoke, such as carbon monoxide are avoided.

Many areas now have smoking cessation support groups and practitioners who have a specific remit for smoking cessation. Contact the local GP surgery, local pharmacy, Health Visiting or Midwifery service for further information. Information leaflets on smoking cessation are available for women and their partners and can be given out during pre-conception and antenatal consultations. The National Institute for Clinical Excellence (NICE) also has guidance on NRT in their *Information for Patients* leaflet (www.nice.org.uk).

It is easy to forget the risks associated with smoking in pregnancy when working with women who are using a whole variety of other drugs. Many women themselves are more concerned about the effects of other drugs, especially opiates. Professionals need to remind themselves that providing information on the risks of smoking is important if they are to convey a balanced and consistent message on the subject.

Advice on alcohol consumption

Safe levels of alcohol use in pregnancy have yet to be precisely established, so ideally women should abstain from alcohol during pregnancy. Alcohol differs from other drugs in that it is generally considered socially acceptable to drink occasionally.

If a pregnant woman chooses not to drink during her pregnancy then she should be encouraged for this decision and not pressured to drink.

The Royal College of Obstetricians and Gynaecologists (RCOG) recommend that pregnant women be advised not to drink more than *one unit of alcohol per day*.[46]

Please note:

One '*unit*' of alcohol is the equivalent to:
- half a pint of 3.5 per cent beer
- one 25 ml measure of spirits

46. Taylor 2003

One small (125ml) glass of average strength (12 per cent) wine contains 1.5 units.

Annex 1 (2003) of the guidelines produced by the Scottish Intercollegiate Guidelines Network, *The Management of Harmful Drinking and Alcohol Dependence in Primary Care*, gives a good detailed information on alcohol unit measures www.sign.ac.uk/pdf/sign74.pdf.

Remember that home measures are often much larger than pub measures. 'Sensible drinking' for women who are *not pregnant* is defined as not consuming more than 3 units in any day (i.e. no more than 21 units per week), and avoiding any heavy 'binge' drinking, defined as consuming double the recommended daily amount on one occasion i.e. 6 units or more for women.

Antenatal screening for problem drinking

It is important that information on alcohol consumption is integrated into routine history taking in antenatal care. Routine antenatal care provides a useful opportunity to *screen* for hazardous levels of drinking and to deliver *brief interventions* for reducing alcohol consumption.[47] **Alcohol use, especially at the level of harmful use, often goes undetected.** Women who drink heavily before conception are more likely to continue drinking heavily during pregnancy without intervention and concurrent drug and alcohol use is associated with poorer outcomes.[48]

It is important that these women are identified early in pregnancy and are offered help, with follow-up through home visits by the community midwife.

There is good evidence that *screening questionnaires* (such as TWEAK, T-ACE or shortened versions of AUDIT) can improve detection of problem drinking in pregnancy and are easy and quick to administer in antenatal and obstetric settings.[49] The Royal College of Obstetricians and Gynaecologists (RCOG) recommends the T-ACE screening test as the most effective way of detecting harmful levels of alcohol consumption in pregnancy.[50] **Routine antenatal screening, using the T-ACE screening test is therefore recommended** (see appendix 5). This simple four-question test that takes about one minute to ask will correctly identify the majority (approximately 70 per cent) of hazardous drinkers during pregnancy. The **T-ACE** questions are listed below.

47. Chang et al 1999
48. Robertson 1998
49. Bradley et al 1998
50. Taylor 2003

T (tolerance)   How many drinks does it take to make you feel high?
Answer: '*3 or more drinks*' scores 2 points

A (annoyance)   Have people annoyed you by criticising your drinking?
Answer: '*Yes*' scores 1 point

C (cut down)   Have you ever felt you ought to cut down your drinking?
Answer: '*Yes*' scores 1 point

E (eye-opener)   Have you ever had a drink first thing in the morning to steady
your nerves or to get rid of a hangover?
Answer: '*Yes*' scores 1 point

A total score of greater than or equal to *two points* is considered positive.

There is also TWEAK, another alcohol questionnaire which is quick to administer
(see appendix 6).

Management of problem alcohol use

Most women will cut down their alcohol consumption when they find out they
are pregnant or when they are given advice to do so. *Brief interventions, harm
reduction advice, motivational interviewing* and *relapse prevention techniques*
are effective methods of reducing low to moderate levels of drinking. For
further information on these interventions see *The Management of Harmful
Drinking and Alcohol Dependence in Primary Care*,[51] and *Brief Interventions*
factsheet.[52]

If a **hazardous drinking score** is obtained using the T-ACE test, check out the
information on www.downyourdrink.org.uk and then professionals should consider
offering the woman one or more of the following interventions:
- Give the woman clear advice to cut down her alcohol consumption
- Ensure the woman is educated about the increased risks associated with
moderate to high levels of drinking in pregnancy
- Complete a *drink diary* (see appendix 7) by asking the woman to detail what
she had to drink on each of the previous seven days
- Ask the woman to describe in more detail her pattern of drinking and alcohol
consumption *before* conception and *since* conception

51. *SIGN guideline 2003*
52. *Alcohol Concern 1997, factsheets 15 (revised 2001), 8, 2 (revised 2004) www.alcoholconcern.org.uk*

- Discuss your concerns with the woman's midwife, consultant obstetrician, GP or other key worker (preferably with the client's consent)
- Arrange an appointment for the woman to see the consultant obstetrician or GP
- Consider referral to an *alcohol service* for specialist assessment and advice (gently broach this subject with her and obtain consent before referral)

Alcohol detoxification

Dependent alcohol use is such a serious risk to the foetus that *detoxification* should be considered at any gestation. Tolerance to alcohol normally develops at high levels of consumption; however tolerance may develop at lower levels of consumption in some women using multiple drugs. Sudden cessation of heavy drinking is potentially dangerous to the mother (because of seizures) and may cause foetal distress. Alcohol dependent pregnant women should be advised *not to* suddenly stop drinking but to consult their GP as soon as possible. Alcohol detoxification requires close monitoring of mother and foetus under specialist medical supervision that includes collaboration with an obstetrician and alcohol specialist and is normally conducted in an inpatient setting.[53] Since the effects of alcohol are associated with dietary deficiencies, the importance of a balanced diet and vitamin supplementation should be discussed. Liver function tests, including prothrombin time should be measured. Disulfiram (*Antabuse*) is *contraindicated* for women who are pregnant or breastfeeding because of the risk of teratogenic effects. Women who conceive whilst taking this drug should receive counselling before deciding to continue with the pregnancy.[54]

Those women who report that they are *unable* to reduce high levels of consumption should be referred to the specialist alcohol services.

Alcohol detoxification should be discussed and agreed with the woman's consultant obstetrician and alcohol specialist beforehand and should be part of a package of care that includes relapse prevention (see section Risk of relapse, page 73).

53. *Plant 2001*
54. *Ibid*

Assessing drug related problems

It is important to establish an accurate picture of a woman's drug use during pregnancy so that appropriate interventions and care can be offered.

An **assessment of drug use** during pregnancy may include such things as:
- taking a detailed history of the woman's drug use
- asking the woman to complete a *drug diary* (see appendix 7)
- assessing drug-related harm (e.g. the physical, psychological, social, legal, financial, lifestyle consequences of the woman's drug use)
- assessing the woman's aspirations and *motivation to change*
- *toxicology* (to screen for recent drug use)
- assessment of *withdrawal* symptoms
- *tolerance testing* or supervised self-administration of methadone

Professionals who are involved in the assessment or care of a woman with a drug related problem should:
- Discuss the woman's care with her General Practitioner or other adviser
- Refer the woman to an appropriate drug service if she is not already attending one so that an assessment can be made
- Seek advice from the woman's drug treatment specialist

Management of problem drug use

The **key aim** of professionals should be to attract women into health and social care treatment services, provide antenatal care and stabilise or reduce drug use to the lowest possible dose.

Much of the skill in drug management lies in planning realistic and achievable goals with each individual woman. Professionals need to be careful not to force their own ideals or 'agenda' on the woman. Many women already feel *guilty* and *worried* about the effects their drug use may be having on their unborn child. If women feel they are not meeting the perceived expectations of professionals they may under-report their drug use and conceal any difficulties they may be experiencing. Trying to persuade a woman to reduce or stop using drugs may simply alienate her, lead to relapse and a sense of failure and result in non-attendance. Different treatment options need to be considered in the light of the woman's aspirations and particular social and psychological circumstances. Drug use may have been an integral part of the woman's lifestyle for many years and she may have no intention of changing this. She may have had a previous pregnancy whilst using drugs with no apparent ill effects. This may be reinforced by drug-using friends who have also successfully delivered healthy babies.[55]

Different **drug treatment options** to consider include:
- Safer drug use advice and education
- Needle exchange and safer injecting advice
- Substitute prescribing
- Stabilisation
- Slow reduction
- Detoxification

Safer drug use

Injecting and *chaotic drug use* in pregnancy is associated with increased risks for both mother and baby. These risks include:
- sudden death through drug *overdose*
- transmission of blood-borne viruses (including HIV, hepatitis C and hepatitis B)
- other complications associated with poor injecting practices and the contaminants contained in non-pharmaceutically prepared street drugs
- pre-term labour and delivery
- multiple social problems

Reducing illicit, chaotic and injecting drug use in pregnancy is therefore an important goal to work towards.

Pregnant women who are injecting drugs can be referred to drug services offering harm reduction facilities: supplies of clean injecting equipment, specialist advice about safer injecting practices and the 'low threshold' methadone programme. Free supplies of clean needles and syringes can be obtained from many pharmacies.

Substitute prescribing

Methadone maintenance is the most generally accepted treatment for opiate dependent pregnant women.[56]

Methadone is normally taken orally in liquid form (methadone mixture 1mg/1ml).

55. Johnstone 1998
56. Kandall et al 1999

It is used to help people *stabilise* their drug intake and associated lifestyle. Because methadone mixture is *long-acting* it offers stability of drug levels for both mother and foetus.

There is *strong research evidence*[57] for the benefits of **methadone maintenance** treatment when given consistently, in adequate dosage, with adequate supervision and in the context of psychosocial support. Five identified benefits according to the research literature[58] include the:

- reduction of injecting behaviour
- reduction of the risk of viral transmission (HIV, hepatitis B and C)
- reduction of drug related deaths
- reduction of illicit drug use
- reduction of offending behaviour

Follow-up studies suggest the long-term outcome in women who enter methadone treatment programmes during pregnancy is better in terms of their pregnancy, childbirth and infant development, irrespective of continued illicit drug use.[59] Women attending treatment services usually have *better antenatal care* and *better general health* than drug-using women *not* in treatment, even if they are still using illicit drugs on top of their substitute prescription.

Dihydrocodeine (DF118) may still be prescribed by some drug treatment services or GPs, it is not universally recommended as the substitute drug of choice for pregnant women. This is due to its shorter half-life and potential for abuse. Information about the use of Buprenorphine (Subutex) in pregnant opioid-dependent women is limited, although the few available case reports have not demonstrated any significant problem. It is more widely used in Austria and France. Research found that methadone and slow-release morphine proved to be safe and efficacious in pregnancy but were found to cause NAS in infants of treated women.[60] Buprenorphine, however, was associated with no or mild NAS. For women who are reluctant to start on methadone, it could provide a useful alternative.

There is also some evidence that babies born to these mothers may be at lower risk of Neonatal Abstinence Syndrome than with other opiates.[61] However it should be noted that the assessment and scoring of NAS may be influenced by the

---

57. *Department of Health 1999*
58. *Ward et al 1998*
59. *Department of Health 1999*
60. *Fischer 1999*
61. *Wright and Walker 2001*

professional's subjective, and often, pejorative view, of drug users in general, and drug-using mothers in particular. Research carried out in Manchester has demonstrated that the appointment of a drug liaison midwife, a robust antenatal assessment and modified scoring system reduced the need of pharmacological intervention by 65 per cent.[62]

Benzodiazepine dependency can be particularly problematic. The treatment approach has changed in recent years due to lack of evidence of its effectiveness and concerns that long-term use may cause cognitive impairment and mood disturbance. Many drug users, however, continue to be prescribed diazepam (Valium). The recommended *maximum* dose of diazepam is now 30mg per day. General Practitioners are advised to reduce doses larger than these and *not* start any new drug user on prescribed benzodiazepines. Women who are prescribed benzodiazepines are normally advised to reduce to the lowest possible dose in pregnancy, and ideally come off completely. Temazepam should **not** be prescribed to pregnant or post-natal women by maternity services for night sedation.

Stabilisation

Pregnant women who are **opiate dependent** *should not* be required to make a commitment to reduce or come off their prescribed opiate drugs. Careful discussion can reassure the woman that being drug-free by the end of the pregnancy is not usually the best option. Indeed it places her in a very vulnerable position, both to the risk of overdose and the stresses of caring for a new baby. The emphasis instead should be on support and engagement rather than enforced reduction or abstinence.[63] Setting individualised goals and stabilising drug use should be the *first priority* and will usually take some time to achieve.

The aim is to *minimise the risks* to mother and baby, not only during pregnancy and the neonatal period, but ideally in the long term. Stable drug use, a stable lifestyle and abstaining from illicit (street) drug use are successful outcomes of treatment.

If non-prescribed opiate use persists, the methadone dose may need to be increased in order to achieve stability and to help the woman abstain from street drug use.[64] However, the risk of overdose if other drugs are taken and the possibility of *Neonatal Abstinence Syndrome* (NAS) need to be understood by the woman (see page 35).

62. D'Souza 2004
63. Wright and Walker 2001
64. Department of Health 1999

Some studies show that plasma levels of methadone *decrease* with gestation.[65] This may be due to the increased fluid space and a large tissue reservoir as well as altered metabolism of the drug by the placenta and foetus. Lowering the dose to avoid complications may therefore be inappropriate and the woman may require an *increase* in methadone during gestation. Advising the woman to try dividing her daily dose can sometimes overcome the need for an increase.[66] Conversely, in the immediate postnatal period, a reversal of these effects may lead to *increased* methadone plasma levels with intoxication effects and the dose may need to be reduced. It is important to warn the woman about this effect as it may have implications for the care and safety of the baby.

Reduction

Slow reduction in pregnancy is also an option but should be gradual, stepwise and tailored to the woman's response. Generally the principle of incremental reductions in drug dosage to a level that minimises withdrawal in the foetus should be explored with the woman. If the woman is dependent on benzodiazepines as well as opiates, then she should be advised to try reducing her **benzodiazepines** first. Diazepam (Valium) is the drug of choice to prescribe, as it is longer acting than other benzodiazepines. Temazepam should be converted to diazepam. **Diazepam** should be prescribed at *no more than* 30mg daily, reducing fortnightly-monthly in 2mg to 5mg decrements. **Methadone** can be reduced weekly or fortnightly in 2.5ml to 5ml decrements.

Dihydrocodeine (DF118) can also be prescribed at *no more than* 30mg tablets x 15 per day, reducing one tablet per week for 15 weeks. Women who are on **buprenorphine** when they become pregnant should be referred for specialist drug management.

As many women will be using more than one substance it is important to address which drug takes priority for reduction. Alcohol, crack cocaine and benzos are top of the list.

Some opiates users may require larger amounts for pain relief as normal doses may be ineffective if tolerance has developed. Drug misuse is **not** a contraindication to having a PCA pump (patient controlled analgesia) following caesarean section and post-delivery pain relief/control should be available as for every woman. However

65. Johnstone 1998
66. Department of Health 1999

it is good practice not to prescribe opiate-based analgesia for routine pain relief, unless absolutely unavoidable, for women who already have a drug dependency.

Detoxification

Detoxification from **opiate** drugs may be considered at any gestation, however it is normally recommended during the second trimester.[67] Rapid detoxification should be avoided in late pregnancy.[68] In the first trimester it is associated with an increased risk of *miscarriage* and in the third trimester it has been associated with *pre-term labour.*[69] Opiate detoxification is rarely fatal for the mother and less serious than withdrawal from benzodiazepines or alcohol, but can be very unpleasant.

Rapid benzodiazepine detoxification should be avoided as this can lead to withdrawal seizures (fits) in the mother and foetal distress.[70] Detoxification treatment should be similar to that of alcohol detoxification. Hospital or residential admission is necessary to supervise a gradual titrated detoxification and to monitor the foetus.

Detoxification should be discussed and agreed with the woman's consultant obstetrician and drug specialist/prescriber beforehand and should be part of a comprehensive package of care that includes relapse prevention.

Over the years, much emphasis has been placed on pregnancy being a *catalyst for change* or a *window of opportunity* for women to either stop using drugs or to reduce their drug use and many pregnant women will tell professionals that this is what they want to do. But experience has shown that this has not generally proved to be the case. Many women who try to reduce or come off drugs during pregnancy are not successful. Maintenance may be more realistic if the woman is trying to become drug-free perhaps for the first time in a long time – and then has to deal with a crying baby. However, all attempts that pregnant women make to improve their health and social circumstances should be supported by professionals and be regarded as a successful outcome of care.

67. *Department of Health 1999*
68. *Johnstone 1998*
69. *Department of Health 1999*
70. *Ibid*

Maternity care

This section provides information and *guidelines on good practice* for maternity care. Maternity care includes:

- pre-conception care
- antenatal care
- intrapartum care
- postnatal care/parenthood

Pre-conception care

Good health and social circumstances *before* pregnancy benefits the woman, her unborn baby and the wider family. All professionals should routinely ask women whether they have any plans to have a child in the near future, or whether they may be currently pregnant. This questioning needs to be done *sensitively* as part of the overall assessment and care planning process. Helping a woman prepare and plan for pregnancy and motherhood provides a good opportunity to offer healthy lifestyle and *harm reduction* education and advice.

All women with drug and alcohol related problems could benefit from receiving information and advice on:

- contraception
- sexual health
- reproductive health
- pre-conception care.

Reproductive health and drug use

Reliable information on how drug use affects women's reproductive health has been difficult to establish and findings are often inconclusive. Theoretically, illicit and dependent drug use can affect fertility in a number of ways.[71]

Substance misuse is associated with poor nutrition and loss of appetite. Significant weight loss can cause *amenorrhoea* (absent periods) with *anovulation* (failure to ovulate or produce eggs).

Opiates (such as heroin, methadone and DF118) and stimulants (such as amphetamines, cocaine and ecstasy) can interfere with a woman's monthly cycle in this way.

71. *Ford and Hepburn 1997*

Amenorrhoea *does not* necessarily mean that the woman is unable to conceive (fall pregnant) as she may still be ovulating, so effective contraception to avoid unwanted pregnancies is still required. Irregular or absent periods means that some women may not realise they are pregnant until late in pregnancy when foetal movements are felt, or until other changes are noticed.

Fertility may increase around the time when a woman reduces or comes off drugs or when she starts treatment with substitute drugs, such as methadone. Offering contraceptive advice and pre-conception counselling therefore needs to go hand in hand with the beginning of any drug treatment.[72]

All professionals can encourage women to attend health care services that provide *contraceptive* and *sexual health* advice and care. GPs and family planning clinics will discuss contraceptive options and advise women about how to get emergency contraception if needed.

Women with substance misuse problems may plan to conceive or may have an unplanned pregnancy. If pregnancy is planned then *pre-conception care* can be offered.

Pre-conception advice

Health, social and voluntary sector professionals all have a role to play in providing pre-conception care to women with substance misuse problems.[73] General Practitioners are in an ideal position to provide pre-conception care to drug-using women who are attending their medical practice for a substitute prescription. If the woman is attending the *Community Drug Team* for her prescription then specialist drug workers have an excellent opportunity to provide pre-conception care. Other workers can address many of the social issues and encourage women to attend to any health checks that they may need.

Pre-conception care may include a discussion on some or all of the following topics:
- Information on local maternity services and the importance of antenatal care
- The woman's past obstetric history, including past pregnancy outcomes and the health and social circumstances of previous children
- The importance of good nutrition and a healthy balanced diet

72. *Ford and Hepburn 1997*
73. *Ibid*

- The use of folic acid to prevent neural tube defects
- Checking for rubella immunity and vaccination if indicated
- Testing for sexually transmitted diseases if needed e.g. chlamydia
- Cervical smear if needed
- Screening for toxoplasmosis and cytomegalovirus (if HIV positive or immunosuppressed)
- The importance of good oral hygiene and dental care
- The benefits of breastfeeding
- Immunisation for hepatitis B, and possibly hepatitis A
- Healthy lifestyle education, including physical exercise, reducing stress etc
- The importance of post-natal contraception and preventing unwanted pregnancies
- Assessment of other physical and psychological health problems that may affect pregnancy and parenthood i.e. significant illnesses, domestic abuse, past or present mental health problems etc
- Assessment of social circumstances, including such issues as housing, debts and welfare benefits, employment and training, offending behaviour and legal circumstances etc
- Assessment of support networks, including partners, parents, other family members and friends
- Previous child protection concerns
- The partner's history of drug/alcohol related problems, including their current use and level of stability if drug dependent
- Advice on relationships and the transition into parenthood
- Advice on child development, parenting skills and information on child care services

Pre-conception advice on drug use can include:
- The risks associated with smoking in pregnancy and information on smoking cessation
- The risks of moderate to excessive alcohol use in pregnancy and advice on how to cut down consumption
- Information on local alcohol services and how to access them
- The risks associated with illicit drug use, in particular injecting drug use
- The risk of Neonatal Abstinence Syndrome (NAS) in babies born to dependent mothers
- Options for drug management in pregnancy and the importance of substitute prescribing and stability for opiate dependent women

- Information on local drug services and how to access them
- Testing for blood borne viruses (HIV, hepatitis C and hepatitis B)
- Information on mother-to-baby transmission of blood-borne viruses and how this can be reduced

All women with a poor obstetric or medical history, or a previous poor foetal or obstetric outcome, or a family history of significant illness should be offered specific pre-conception services. The woman should be encouraged to discuss this with her General Practitioner in the first instance.

Antenatal care

Receiving good quality antenatal care is known to improve pregnancy outcomes, irrespective of continued drug/alcohol use. **All women with substance misuse problems should be told about the benefits of antenatal care and advised to attend early in pregnancy.**

Maternity care in the UK is now essentially community based and midwife managed unless there are particular complications that necessitate obstetric-led care. Both GPs and midwives are able to discuss what care options are available in the area where the woman lives. Home delivery is not generally considered to be a suitable option for drug using women, usually because of the potential for NAS in the newborn. However in Manchester for example, several women have had uncomplicated home deliveries following careful assessment of suitability. A priority is to ensure a robust risk assessment regarding venous access is completed for those with a history of injecting. Increased daily visits post-natally by a supportive community midwife and specialist midwife will offer additional support to the few women who request or insist on a home delivery.

Community midwives and GPs now successfully manage the majority of pregnant women with substance misuse problems. Many areas also now have designated specialist midwives, often jointly employed by drug and maternity services, who co-ordinate care and provide extra input for women with alcohol and drug misuse. Multi-agency case planning ensures all relevant information is shared, particularly if there are Child Protection concerns. Sharing information amongst practitioners working with children and families is essential. In many cases it is only when information from a range of sources is put together that a child can be seen to be in need, many families will require help and support.

All pregnant women receive a copy of the *Pregnancy Book,* produced by the Department of Health. It contains comprehensive information on all aspects of pregnancy, childbirth and postnatal care and will help the woman in her decision-making. The GP will normally give a copy of the book to the woman at confirmation of pregnancy or the midwife will give it to her at booking.

Hand held maternity records

All pregnant women carry their own *woman-held* maternity record. This is normally given to the woman at the booking appointment and she keeps it until the baby is born. The woman is encouraged to contribute to her notes if she wishes. **Record keeping is an integral part of care.** All professionals involved in a woman's care should ensure that important information is put in writing and included in the woman's maternity record.

The 'booking appointment'

Pregnant women can self refer to a midwife, be referred by their GP or other agency. The *booking appointment* is normally arranged for 12 weeks gestation and is a very important appointment for the woman to attend. A dating scan at this stage is very helpful in assessing the ongoing growth of the baby. At the booking appointment the midwife completes a *comprehensive assessment* of the woman's needs and will plan pregnancy care with the woman. The midwife also undertakes a *risk assessment* to take into account any factors that might affect pregnancy outcome and the woman's ability to care for her baby. All women receive their care in the community unless they have been identified as 'high risk', in which case they will have their care managed by a Consultant Obstetrician who may arrange for their care to be delivered in the hospital.

At the booking appointment the midwife routinely asks about all drug use, including smoking, alcohol use, illicit drug use and prescribed drug use. Drug taking details are recorded in the woman's hand held maternity record, unless she requests otherwise.

It is important to remember that for some women their drug and alcohol use may come to light for the first time because of their pregnancy care. If this happens it is an excellent opportunity to offer **harm reduction advice** and education and it may lead to a change in the woman's drug use. Other women may know they have a drug or alcohol related problem but choose *not to disclose* this information to health and social care professionals. Some women may acknowledge that they use alcohol or drugs but grossly under-report their use. These women are sometimes identified when problems manifest in the neonate, a which point help can be offered.

Many women with drug related problems would already be known to drug services and be already on prescribed medication. Sharing information is vital to ensure a streamlined service where there is no duplication or ambiguity in either prescribing or advice.

Routine antenatal screening at booking

At the booking appointment, the community midwife will also offer *routine antenatal screening*. Blood samples are taken for: HIV, hepatitis B, rubella, syphilis, blood group and a full blood count.

Please note the following regarding **blood-borne viruses**:
- Women who are currently injecting drugs or who have a history of *injecting drug use* may be at risk of HIV, hepatitis B and hepatitis C.
- The hepatitis B *vaccine* can be given safely in pregnancy and should be offered to all women who are likely to inject drugs in pregnancy or whose partner is an injecting drug user.
- The Hepatitis C antibody test is *not* offered routinely as part of antenatal care, however it *should* be offered to all pregnant women at risk.
- Many women who use drugs may *not* have a history of injecting themselves, but may have a *partner who does*.
- Non-drug using women may be at risk of blood borne virus infection if they have *unprotected sex* with an infected man.

For more detailed information on **antenatal testing for HIV, hepatitis B and C** and the **management of positive women and their babies** see appendix 1.

Other screening and diagnostic tests

Numerous screening and diagnostic procedures are offered during pregnancy. These are especially important for drug and alcohol using women who may be at increased risk of pregnancy complications. Drug use is associated with an increased risk of **intrauterine growth restriction (IUGR)** so care should be taken to assess foetal growth by clinical examination, ultrasound and antenatal foetal monitoring. Tobacco is a causal factor in IUGR, and it is well documented that the majority of drug users are smokers. Staff should be careful to explain the reasons for any additional tests sensitively to the woman.

Ultrasound scan is normally arranged for 10–14 weeks. It is important partly to confirm gestational age, but also to provide the mother with a positive experience of the hospital. Substance-misusing women often worry about foetal abnormality more than any other problem and feel guilty about the damage they may have caused their baby. In general, it is usually possible to be quite reassuring.[74] Detailed **foetal anomaly scanning** is not normally required as substance misuse is not associated with an increased risk of structural foetal abnormality. The only exceptions would be with heavy alcohol consumption (>6 units/day).

Attendance for **foetal monitoring** (cardiotocography or CTG) may sometimes be necessary for substance-misusing women, particularly if growth restriction (IUGR) is established. Please note however that there may be reduced activity (loss of variability and accelerations) following ingestion of opiates, benzodiazepines and alcohol. Repeat or extended monitoring is sometimes required. The **biophysical profile** is less affected and will usually be normal even after ingestion of drugs. Another foetal monitoring test, the **umbilical artery doppler** assessment, can identify vascular problems in the placenta, which can lead to distress or death. This test might be necessary for women who are heavy users of stimulant drugs (such as cocaine or amphetamines) or women in whom IUGR is demonstrated by ultrasound.

Some women drug users (for instance those working in the sex industry) are at higher risk of **sexually transmitted and other vaginal infections**. Because infections are a risk factor in pre-term labour and delivery it is important to detect and treat all infections in pregnancy. Screening for chlamydia, gonorrhoea, bacterial vaginosis and Group B streptococcus should be considered.

Some women (in particular HIV positive and immuno-compromised women) may also be at greater risk of **cervical intraepithelial neoplasia (CIN)** and may not have attended for routine cytological screening (cervical smears). Pregnancy can be a good opportunity to attract women into cytological surveillance, certainly in the first and early second trimester.

74. Johnstone 1998

Pregnancy complications

Other complications can occur in substance-using women but not much more frequently than other women, with the exception of women using large amounts of stimulants, such as cocaine.[75]

Pre-term labour is a particular problem that poses a difficult start to mothering and is a significant risk to the baby. It is more common in drug dependent women, particularly those using drugs intravenously or taking short-acting opiates (i.e. heroin). Very pre-term delivery is associated with increased mortality. **Infections** also account for some pre-term labour episodes so screening is advisable. Pregnant women should be advised to present themselves *early* if they think they are in pre-term labour so that an injection of steroids can be given to help mature the foetal lungs.

Maternal health problems

Good nutrition in pregnancy is important for the development of the baby. All pregnant women should be given advice about eating a **healthy balanced diet**. Pregnant women are routinely tested for **anaemia** at their antenatal appointments and will be prescribed iron if necessary. They are advised to take **folic acid** for the first 12 weeks of pregnancy to prevent neural tube defects. **Constipation** is very common in pregnancy and can be exacerbated by opiate use, so women should be advised to increase their fibre intake and drink more water.

Poor general health and drug use can lead to **respiratory problems**, including chest infections and asthma. Repeated injections over years destroys peripheral veins, often leaving 'track marks' so **venous access** may be limited even in women who stopped injecting drugs years before.

Good **dental care** in pregnancy is especially important. All pregnant women with substance misuse problems should be encouraged to attend their dentist for a check up so that they can get any necessary dental treatment and avoid dental decay and infections in pregnancy. Severe dental problems are commonly associated with opiate use. This is made worse by the high sugar content and acidity of **methadone.** *Sugar free* methadone is available on prescription, but the acid content is similar to the normal preparation. Advise all women to brush their

75. Johnstone 1998

teeth with fluoride toothpaste *before* they take their methadone and rinse their mouth afterwards with water. Sugar free chewing gum will also help clear the methadone from their mouths. Women tend to suffer increased gum problems during pregnancy, which can show itself as bleeding gums. This can be more serious in women with substance misuse problems and progress to acute and very painful infections.

Benefits and allowances

All pregnant women should be given information on *benefits and allowances* that are available during and after pregnancy. These include:
- Entitlement to **free NHS prescriptions** throughout pregnancy and for one year after the birth of their baby
- Entitlement to **free NHS dental treatment** throughout pregnancy and for one year after the birth of their baby
- The **Sure Start Maternity Grant** (which is currently worth £500 and can be claimed from the 29th week of pregnancy). A midwife, health visitor or doctor will need to sign this form (which confirms that the woman has received health education and antenatal care).
- Entitlement to **free milk** tokens after the birth of their baby

Further information on benefits is available from the Department of Work and Pension www.dwp.gov.uk and the **Social Security Office booklet** *Babies and Children: A basic guide to benefits and tax credits for anyone expecting a baby or caring for children* (BC1 April 2004). Copies of the booklet are available from local Job Centres.

Preparation for parenthood

All pregnant women and their partners are offered 'parent education' and this normally starts at around 32 weeks gestation. Group and individual sessions are organised and run jointly by midwives and health visitors. Parent education is especially important for women with substance misuse problems and for first time mothers and fathers. All parent education sessions are community-based. For further information contact the local Community Midwifery Team. Professionals should encourage parents to attend these sessions as many people with substance misuse problems have not had positive parenting role models and attendance is often poor.

Risk assessment during pregnancy

All professionals working with pregnant women with substance misuse problems should have a clear understanding of the concept of *risk assessment* to ensure **safety for mother and baby**. Risk should be **continuously** assessed throughout the pregnancy, taking into account that risk status is dynamic and may change over time.

Significant **risk factors** that would warrant further assessment and intervention would include:
● Poor obstetric and pregnancy outcome history
● Poor maternal health/significant illness/HIV, Hepatitis C or B
● High alcohol consumption or alcohol dependence
● Injecting drug use or chaotic illicit (non-prescribed) drug use
● Neonate at risk of developing Neonatal Abstinence Syndrome (NAS), or previous baby with NAS
● History of severe mental health problem (e.g. schizophrenia, bipolar disorder, postnatal depression/puerperal psychosis, eating disorder)
● Domestic abuse
● Homelessness and insecure/unsuitable/unsafe accommodation
● Other significant social problems (e.g. legal, financial, unsupported pregnancy, chaotic lifestyle)
● Existing children on 'at risk' register/accommodated by local authority
● Recorded history of previous parenting or child care concerns
● Prostitution

Homelessness

It is important that a homeless woman finds suitable accommodation in time for her to prepare for the birth of her baby. Homelessness creates additional stress for the women and can make attendance for antenatal care difficult. Good liaison and care planning are required to ensure agencies are working together. Pregnant women also need to engage early with the Health Visiting service who will encourage the family to move towards accessing mainstream services once they are in stable accommodation.

Not registered with a GP

Pregnant women who are not registered with a General Practitioner should be encouraged to do so as soon as possible. If the woman experiences any difficulty registering with a GP then she should be advised to contact her Primary Care Trust or call NHS Direct on 0845 4647 to request a GP be allocated to her. Requests must be made in writing. Advise the woman to complete the *proforma* letter (see appendix 4) and send to their local Health Care Services.

Domestic abuse

Pregnancy can of itself be a catalyst for domestic abuse or may escalate during pregnancy. It is a child protection issue.

Domestic abuse can have a harmful, sometimes even life threatening, impact on the physical and mental well being of both mother and baby and is a serious criminal, social and medical problem. Domestic abuse can include a wide range of *physical* (e.g. hitting, kicking, restraining), *sexual* (including rape and coercion), *psychological* (verbal bullying, undermining, social isolation) and *financial* (e.g. withholding money) abuses. Domestic abuse is widespread and under reported and the level of repeat incidence is high. *Conclusive evidence has demonstrated that pregnancy, far from being a time of peace and safety, may trigger or exacerbate male violence in the home.*[76] Violence may also increase following the birth of a child or when a woman tries to end a relationship. All midwives should sensitively enquire about domestic abuse as part of their antenatal risk assessment. Relevant addresses and telephone numbers should be made easily accessible to enable women to get help with or without the support and knowledge of health and social care staff. Women who disclose domestic abuse should be given advice and support on how and where to get help.

Neonate at risk of Neonatal Abstinence Syndrome (NAS)

It is important to discuss at an early stage with all drug dependent women the possibility of *Neonatal Abstinence Syndrome* (NAS). She needs to know that NAS is usually easily managed but the baby will need her support, understanding and patience. Having a baby who develops severe withdrawal symptoms can be very distressing for parents, but if properly looked after the baby will make a full recovery and will come to no short-term developmental harm.[77]

76. *Royal College of Midwives 1997*
77. *Johnstone 1998*

A **parent information leaflet** called *Caring for a baby with drug withdrawal symptoms* is available with this book (see appendix 11). This leaflet should be given to all drug dependent women and their partners at around 32 weeks gestation. They should be advised to read the leaflet and discuss their birth plan and care of their baby with the midwife.

Child care risk

Occasionally, a risk assessment will identify concerns about the ability of the woman (or her partner) to look after their (currently unborn) child. If this is the case, then it is important to address these concerns with the woman at an early stage. All professionals in contact with pregnant women have a responsibility to act if they believe that the baby's safety or welfare will be at significant risk of harm. A pro-active and **early intervention** approach is more likely to result in a positive outcome for both mother and baby.

Professionals should make themselves familiar with their local area child protection guidelines in addition to the following documents:

- **Hidden Harm: Responding to the needs of children of problem drug users** (ACMD report 2003)
- **Every Child Matters** (The Stationery Office 2003)
- **Getting our Priorities Right: Good Practice Guidance for Working with Children and Families Affected by Substance Misuse** (ACMD Report 2003)

These documents contain important information for professionals, including:

- The guiding principles of child protection
- The legal framework on child protection
- Professional roles and responsibilities in relation to protecting the welfare of children
- Guidance on information sharing and confidentiality
- The signs and symptoms of physical abuse, neglect, non organic failure to thrive, emotional abuse and sexual abuse
- The impact of parental problem drug use on infants and children
- The referral process for dealing with child care concerns and child protection
- A checklist of information to be collated concerning substance misuse and its impact on parenting
- The practicalities of protecting and supporting the children of problem drug users

Intrapartum care (labour and childbirth)

The vast majority of labours and deliveries will be straightforward in drug and alcohol using women and thus their care will be similar to any other woman.[78] There are however, a few important factors to consider and guidelines may vary locally.

For instance, currently, intrapartum care in Lothian is provided by labour suite midwives and community midwives who staff the labour suite on rotation. The pregnant woman may see a number of different midwives if she has several antenatal episodes in the labour suite (for instance for pre-term labour) and her key midwife in the community may not be the one who delivers her baby.

The Obstetrician and Paediatrician are kept informed during labour, but they are not the key professionals unless there are complications (for instance, pre-term delivery).

Midwives delivering intrapartum care should make sure they read the woman's *hand held records* and any other important information. For example the **antenatal liaison form (substance misuse)** produced by NHS Lothian, included in this book provides detailed information on the woman's drug/alcohol use, medication, pharmacist and key professionals and services involved in her care (see appendix 8).

Maternity hospital policy

The woman, her partner and family all need to understand the hospital priority for a safe pregnancy and childbirth experience. This means zero tolerance of illicit drug use on hospital premises, clear limits on the number and conduct of herself and any visitors, and zero tolerance for abusive, threatening or aggressive behaviour. If necessary, visitors will be removed from the building and barred from returning.

Substitute prescribed drugs are dispensed by the hospital pharmacy but only after the dose of medication has been checked with the prescribing doctor and any community prescriptions have been cancelled with the pharmacist.

78. Johnstone 1998

This means that hospital staff will need to know the name and telephone number of the *prescribing doctor* and *pharmacy*. This information should be written clearly in the woman's notes. The woman should remember to take any supply of medication into hospital with her, *as it will not be replaced* if it has already been dispensed in the community. On discharge, the hospital will notify the prescribing doctor when the next dose of medication is due to be dispensed from the community.

Pain relief during childbirth

Women who use drugs may be fearful of labour and childbirth and worry that they will not get adequate pain relief. *It is very important that adequate pain relief is given* and the midwife establishes a good rapport with the woman, offering reassurance and support when required. It is a good idea to discuss pain relief options in the *antenatal* period so that the woman feels confident that she will be well cared for and treated like any other woman in labour.

Prescribed medication should be dispensed *as normal* during labour. **Substitution treatment with methadone does not provide pain relief.** Opioid receptors may be saturated so higher doses or more frequent injections of diamorphine are likely to be needed.[79] There is usually a low threshold for an *epidural* anaesthesia and many drug dependent women opt for this pain management approach.

Caesarean section is no more likely than in the normal population and having a history of drug misuse should not be considered a contraindication to having a PCA pump (patient controlled analgesia pump) following caesarean section.[80] Post delivery pain relief should be the same as for every other woman, although higher doses may be required.

Complications of childbirth

In women with a history of injecting drug use, **venous access** may be poor and antenatal referral to an anaesthetist may be required. Where labour is straightforward, no intravenous line is required. However, if it appears that there might be complications, it is sometimes better to establish an intravenous line *electively* shortly after admission, rather than be faced with the task in an emergency situation.[81]

79. *Sparey and Wilkinshaw 1999*
80. *Siney 1999*

There may be **placental insufficiency** in pregnancies of drug-using women, leading to an increased risk of intrapartum hypoxia, foetal distress and meconium staining.[82] **Meconium aspiration** is common and is associated with foetal distress secondary to periods of intra-uterine drug withdrawal. Some babies will be **growth restricted** so there should be careful surveillance during labour. Maternity staff should follow hospital guidelines for obstetric and neonate management for *meconium staining*.

High dose benzodiazepine use in the mother can result in the newborn showing *signs of intoxication* at birth that include: poor sucking, poor reflexes, hypotonia (low muscle tone), hypothermia (low body temperature), a feeble cry and low APGAR scores. Severely affected neonates may require vigorous resuscitation at birth because of respiratory depression. Women who are anxious about childbirth should be warned not to 'self medicate' with non-prescribed benzodiazepines (e.g. Valium) before they admit themselves for delivery.

Please note: Labour ward staff **must not use naloxone** (an opiate antagonist) to reverse opioid induced respiratory depression in neonates as this will induce an abrupt opiate withdrawal crisis. Use supportive measures or ventilation if necessary. Should the baby collapse at birth, this is not usually associated with maternal use of drugs and normal resuscitation procedures would apply.

Postpartum care in hospital

After delivery, the labour ward midwife should liaise with staff in the postnatal ward to ensure continuity of care. The *key midwife* in the community should also be informed of the delivery. This is particularly important if the woman has delivered pre-term. Procedures may vary locally, in Lothian, for instance Maternity staff providing intrapartum care complete the **pregnancy outcome form (substance misuse)** (see appendix 8).

All known drug dependent women are asked to stay in hospital for three days **(72 hours)** following the birth of their baby. This is because the baby needs to be observed for signs and symptoms of **Neonatal Abstinence Syndrome (NAS)**, which normally develop within this time period. However NAS can be delayed for up to 7–10 days if the woman is taking methadone in conjunction with benzodiazepines.

81. Johnstone 1998
82. Department of Health 1999

Confinement in hospital can be a threatening experience for some drug-using women.[83] Staff should take care to *ensure privacy* by being discreet about the administration of any medications (e.g. methadone) so that the woman's drug use is not exposed to other patients or visiting relatives who might not know about her drug use.

Soon after delivery, mother and baby should be transferred to the **postnatal ward** where they can *room in* together and have *skin-to-skin* contact. Separating mother and baby should be avoided if at all possible. *Skin-to-skin* contact will help the baby relax and sleep, regulate their body temperature, steady their breathing, help with mother-infant bonding and will help get breastfeeding off to a good start.

Women who have a history of alcohol related problems (who remain in the postnatal ward) can be observed for maternal symptoms of **alcohol withdrawal** (which typically occur around 48 hours post delivery), in which case appropriate medication may be required.[84]

Ideally, discussion about the need for **postnatal contraception** should have been instigated in the antenatal period rather than at the post-delivery meeting before discharge from hospital. Many women with substance misuse problems are not able to address their reproductive and sexual health care needs adequately.

Planning contraception for the postnatal period involves considering 'what, how and when?' to start using hormonal treatments (e.g. combined oral contraceptive pill, progestogen-only pill, Depo-Provera, Implanon etc) or the coil. Advice on choices also varies depending on whether the woman is breastfeeding or not. Condoms are normally recommended for the first 48 hours post-delivery or for the first few weeks following delivery until hormonal contraception has been started.

After 72 hours on the postnatal ward, mother and baby can be safely **discharged** home, provided the baby is well enough. On discharge, all women should be given a *discharge pack* which contains helpful information leaflets on caring for their baby.

In circumstances where the mother insists on taking an early discharge, she should be seen by the paediatrician and asked to sign a form that states she is taking the

83. Mounteney 1999
84. Wright and Walker 2001

baby home *against medical advice.* But this is not legally binding. In rare cases, the mother may take her own discharge and leave the baby in hospital. If this happens, the baby will be transferred to the Neonatal Unit for continued monitoring.

Infant feeding

Much confusion surrounds the issue of whether a woman should breast feed her baby whilst continuing to take drugs. Many women and their partners are concerned about breastfeeding whilst taking drugs or drinking alcohol and will ask for advice. Parents should be informed that the benefits of breastfeeding *far outweigh* the disadvantages, even with continued drug use. It is important to reassure the mother that the actual amount of most drugs passed to the baby through breast milk is minimal and will have little effect on the newborn baby. The sometimes small effect on the baby may even help withdrawal symptoms, if they are present.

It is important that the woman is not given contradictory advice from different professionals, as nothing is more certain to reduce her confidence and to confuse her decision-making.

Breastfeeding

Breastfeeding should be **encouraged** in drug-using women.[85] Mothers who are on prescribed drugs should therefore be encouraged to breast feed in the same way as other mothers. The exceptions to this would be if she were:
● HIV positive (because of the risk of transmission)
● using large quantities of stimulant drugs, such as cocaine, crack or amphetamines (because of vasoconstriction effects)
● drinking heavily (>6 units/day) or taking large amounts of non-prescribed benzodiazepines (because of sedation effects)

Breastfeeding is best done immediately *before* taking medication and should be avoided for one to two hours after any dose of medication (i.e. the time of highest plasma concentrations). Medications are best taken as a single dose where possible and should be administered before the baby's longest sleep period.[86]

Women who are **Hepatitis B positive** can also safely breastfeed as soon as their newborn baby has had their first dose of immunoglobulin and Hep B vaccine (administered soon after birth).

There is no evidence that hepititic C transmission occurs through breastfeeding and hepatitis C mothers should not be advised against breastfeeding.[87]

85. Department of Health 1999
86. SIGN Postnatal Depression *guideline 2003*
87. Department of Health 2004

Injecting drug use whilst breastfeeding should be discouraged because of the risk of mother-to-baby HIV transmission.

Ideally the woman should keep her drug use as **stable** as possible whilst breastfeeding. Ability to successfully breastfeed is in itself an indication of stability.[88] Breastfeeding can support the mother in feeling that she is positively comforting and caring for her baby and it can aid in the bonding process. Breastfeeding will also benefit the long-term health of both mother and baby.

The benefits of breastfeeding are outlined in the UNICEF leaflet *Feeding Your New Baby*, which mothers-to-be should be given in the antenatal period. For more detailed information about breastfeeding see *Breastfeeding* available from the Department of Health.[89]

Midwives can also offer a great deal of support and advice to mothers who wish to breastfeed their baby. For instance, they show the mother how to position their baby for feeding and how to make sure the baby attaches properly to the breast. They also teach mothers how to recognise when their baby is feeding properly and when not. Most regions across the country have breastfeeding support groups and antenatal breastfeeding workshops. Contact the local Midwifery Team or Health Visiting office for further information on these.

Weaning

The World Health Organisation (WHO 2001) recommends that babies should be exclusively breast fed until about 6 months of age in order to achieve optimal growth, development and health. After 6 months of age, the mother can introduce appropriate solid foods whilst continuing to breastfeed for up to 2 years or beyond.

Formula (bottle) feeds are not a necessary part of a weaning diet. However, if a breastfeeding mother wishes to combine formula feeding with breastfeeding or to switch to formula feeding *she should do this gradually*, substituting one formula feed for one breast feed per day for several days, allowing her baby and her body to become accustomed to this. A second formula feed can then be introduced for another few days, then a third, fourth etc. Ideally, the weaning process should take several weeks, allowing a slow withdrawal for the baby.

---

88. *Hepburn 1996*
89. *You can download the document from www.breatfeeding.nhs.uk or call 08701 555455 quoting reference/Breastfeeding31636*

Abrupt cessation of breastfeeding may result in the baby showing some signs and symptoms of drug withdrawal. Advise breastfeeding mothers who continue to take drugs to gradually introduce solids slowly into the breastfeeding schedule, reducing the frequency of breast feeds over a number of weeks.

Bottle feeding

Many women drug users choose to bottle feed rather than breast feed. Social and cultural beliefs and norms are powerful influences on decision making about early infant feeding. Parents should be supported to make an informed choice about how to feed their newborn baby. Having made their decision, they should be supported by all professionals involved.

Postnatal care

The care of a pregnant woman who uses drugs or alcohol and the safe delivery of her baby is just the start of care. **Continuing support in the postnatal period and for parenthood is essential if the ideal outcome of maintaining a healthy mother and child together is to be achieved.**

After discharge from hospital, the baby is cared for at home by the mother and family, with advice and support from the Community Midwife as well as other professionals and agencies involved with the family. The midwife will visit the family at home each day until the baby is 10 days old. Occasionally the midwife may need to continue visiting up until the baby is 28 days old, depending on how well the baby is and how well the mother is coping. The Health Visitor normally visits after day 10 and should liaise with the midwife and GP before visiting the family. The Health Visitor will be a good source of information and support on motherhood and all aspects of health for the woman and her baby. When the baby is 6–8 weeks old, the GP and Health Visitor will arrange a comprehensive postnatal examination of mother and baby.

Postnatal care should facilitate women and their partners to make an effective **transition into parenthood**. Professionals should give women and their partners an opportunity to reflect on their experiences of pregnancy and childbirth in the postnatal period as well as an opportunity to discuss the effects of parenthood on their relationships.

Soon after mother and baby are home, a **case discussion meeting** should be organised by the lead professional to review the care plan and to decide whether an appropriate level of support is in place for the family.

Postnatal depression

Women drug users may be more at risk of *postnatal depression* and other mental health problems. Anxiety, depression and a history of sexual and/or physical abuse are commonly associated with drug and alcohol dependency. Identifying, screening and supporting women at risk of postnatal depression is very important. Untreated postnatal depression is associated with detrimental effects on infant development. Many Primary Care Trusts are now addressing Postnatal Depression in their Health Improvement Plans. Improved maternal and child mental health are key objectives of the SureStart programmes.

Postnatal depression can be assessed using the *Edinburgh Postnatal Depression Score* (EPDS) screening tool and augmented by a multi-disciplinary *Integrated Care Pathways* (ICP). Health Visitors and GPs are trained to use these tools to improve the care of women at risk. Staff should make themselves familiar with relevant guidelines.

Sudden Infant Death Syndrome (SIDS)

Maternal tobacco use, as well as drug and alcohol misuse are associated with an increased risk of *Sudden Infant Death Syndrome* (SIDS or cot death). All parents who use these drugs should be given advice about how to *reduce the risk* of cot death. The leaflet 'Reducing the risk of cot death' (produced by the Department of Health) should be included in the hospital discharge pack.

Risk of relapse

In the postnatal period, increased drug and alcohol use is common. For women who have managed to reduce their intake during pregnancy or even come off drugs or alcohol, the risk of relapse to former levels of drug taking is high. There are a number of reasons for this, including:

- feeling that it's now OK to use again
- relief at having a 'normal' baby
- wanting to celebrate!
- the stress of caring for a new born baby (perhaps with NAS)

- 'baby blues' or postnatal depression
- poor support from partner or family
- anxieties about motherhood

It is important for professionals to acknowledge that relapse is common. Re-assessment of substance use and *careful drug management* is essential at this time, along with support to remain stable and to prevent relapse.

Ensuring the woman is engaged with a specialist drug and alcohol agency that can provide a relapse prevention service may be an *important part* of the postnatal care plan.

Relapse prevention support work can include:
- helping parents understand relapse as a process and as an event
- raising awareness of 'high-risk' situations and factors that might lead to relapse
- exploration of how to anticipate, avoid or cope with these high-risk situations
- acquisition of skills (cognitive and behavioural) to implement relapse prevention strategies
- anxiety and stress management education
- confidence building and improving self–efficacy
- strengthening existing positive coping strategies and other personal attributes
- life/social skills education (e.g. assertiveness, resistance and dissuasion skills, alternative activities to drug/alcohol use)

Assessing and managing child care risk during pregnancy

Many pregnant women who have substance misuse problems worry that they will be referred to social services or their baby will be taken into care purely because they use drugs. Raising this subject early and discussing their concerns openly will foster a more trusting relationship. **It is important to reassure women that substance misuse, in itself, is not sufficient reason to assume inadequate parenting or child care.** They need to know, however, that if there are specific concerns about the safety or welfare of the child then social work may need to do an assessment and get involved, but that this policy is the same for everyone, whether or not they use drugs. This advice is mentioned in the information leaflet *Pregnant... and using drugs or alcohol?* (see appendix 10).

Many different factors affect the health and development of children. Parental drug and alcohol use is just one factor. Research evidence *does not* support the assumption that parental substance misuse will automatically lead to child neglect or abuse.[90] Indeed, a number of *case controlled studies* in Britain have found no significant differences in the health and development of children in drug-using households compared to non-drug using households.[91] Becoming 'drug free' should not be a requirement for parents to keep their children living with them. Parents who stop using drugs or control their drug intake are not necessarily better or safer parents. Some parents will have poor parenting skills for reasons other than their substance misuse as many risk factors also occur in non-drug using families.

However, a chaotic drug or alcohol using lifestyle *may* affect child safety and the child's health and development in a number of ways and is always a factor to be considered. Infants, in particular, are vulnerable to the effects of physical and emotional neglect or injury which can have damaging effects on their long-term development.

A number of **childcare problems** have been associated with parental substance misuse.[92] Some of these include:

- Inconsistent caring
- Inadequate supervision
- Lack of stimulation
- Inadequate and unsafe accommodation
- Social isolation and stigma
- Exposure to violence and criminal behaviour

---

90. *Scottish Executive 2003*
91. *Ross et al 1995, Burns et al 1996*
92. *Scottish Executive 2003, ACMD 2003*

- Emotional or physical neglect or abuse

Resulting in ...
- Failure to thrive
- Accidental injury
- Emotional difficulties
- Behavioural difficulties
- Poor social development
- Poor cognitive and educational attainment

Professionals who are involved with children and families need to remember that good **inter-agency communication** and **collaboration** in the care process is essential. It is important to **obtain consent** from the woman early to share information with other professionals and agencies (see consent form in appendix 3). No professional, however, can guarantee absolute confidentiality as both statute and common law accepts that information may be shared in certain circumstances.

Childcare risk assessment should cover issues such as existing parenting skills, child safety, as well as the physical, cognitive, emotional and social development of children. Drug and alcohol specialist workers that lack child care and parenting expertise should consult with and involve other professionals and agencies who do have this expertise.

The Scottish Executive (2003) document *Getting Our Priorities Right: Good practice Guidance for working with Children and Families affected by Substance Misuse,* appendix II, includes a helpful **checklist** for collating information on substance misuse and its impact on parenting (download from www.scotland.gov.uk). See also *Every Child Matters* (The Stationery Office 2003, download from www.rcu.gov.uk/articles/news/everychildmatters.pdf).

The assessment process may highlight **concerns** because the woman or her partner:
- has a very chaotic lifestyle with multiple social problems and repeatedly fails to attend antenatal appointments
- attends appointments but are repeatedly intoxicated or incapacitated from the effects of alcohol or drugs
- has an inappropriate home environment which could be unsafe for a baby
- lacks the necessary material possessions for caring for a baby
- has been previously referred to social work regarding their parenting ability

- has existing children on the child protection register
- has had previous children accommodated by the local authority
- has had previous children adopted
- discloses domestic abuse
- is socially isolated with no support network
- engages in 'disguised compliance' where she pre-empts home visits by coming to the service to keep professionals at arms length from the home.

Child protection

The welfare of the child is the paramount consideration. All professionals working with pregnant women and families affected by substance misuse should make themselves familiar with their local area child protection guidelines.

Professionals who have concerns could consider taking one or more of the following **actions**:

- Refer to a **non-statutory service** that works with children and families affected by substance misuse. Substance-misusing parents see non-statutory services as more acceptable and less 'stigmatising' than social work. Professionals who work in these services can offer intensive parenting support.
- Discuss your concerns with the Midwife, Health Visitor or General Practitioner
- Contact your designated senior staff member with responsibility for child protection to discuss your concerns
- Contact your local duty social work service (Children and Families Team) to discuss your concerns and to seek their advice
- Encourage the woman to approach social services herself for help and advice

If there is a **significant risk of harm** to the baby's health and development then **professionals should take action** and refer to social services. Significant harm may result from maltreatment or the absence of adequate care. The protection of children is an interagency responsibility, but **social work** has a statutory responsibility to assess risk and ensure that child protection plans are in place if necessary. The social work assessment, while acknowledging the needs and the rights of the parents, will focus primarily on the *needs and welfare of the child*. In some situations there will be conflict between the needs and wishes of the parents and the welfare of the child.

Any referral or discussion with social services should be **handled sensitively**. It is important to stress to the woman that social work involvement is often positive and helpful. Whenever possible, social work has a duty to promote children's upbringing by their families. Compulsory removal of children from their families is rare, even when agencies are worried about a child's welfare.

Occasionally, social services will be sufficiently concerned about the future risk to an unborn child to warrant the implementation of **child protection procedures** and the calling of a **child protection case conference** to consider the need for registration and a child protection plan. If a *child protection case conference* is called, ideally it should be held 6–8 weeks before the estimated delivery date so that services can be put in place in time for the birth of the baby.

Early intervention strategies

For families who are of *concern* but not formally *at risk*, professionals should take the opportunity to engage with the parents and **intervene early**. A range of interventions can be helpful for pregnant women and vulnerable children and families. These include offering **parenting support** by:

- Offering emotional support and an opportunity to talk about any stresses or worries
- Discussing parenting roles and responsibilities
- Developing the parents existing skills, attributes and resources
- Promoting a safer and more stable lifestyle
- Teaching strategies to develop good parent/infant bonding
- Offering or arranging practical support to the family
- Teaching good play techniques and parent/child activities
- Discussing strategies for managing their children's behaviour
- Engaging them in activities where they can experience positive role modelling
- Helping parents develop routines, guidelines and boundaries with their children

Protective factors

Professionals who provide care to pregnant women and their partners can ensure that **protective factors in child welfare are promoted** by *routinely* discussing the following topics both *before* and *after* the baby is born:

Drug safety issues in the home ... safe storage of drugs, safe storage and disposal of injecting equipment, risks of ingestion of drugs and overdose, how to deal with medical emergencies etc

The importance of providing for all the child's basic needs ... food, clothes, warmth, personal hygiene, comfort, safety, stimulation, age-appropriate activities etc

The importance of attending any child health appointments with the doctor and Health Visitor

The importance of providing appropriate supervision for their children ... periods of intoxication and withdrawal may be a time when adequate supervision cannot be provided and parents will need to ensure that another responsible adult is available in these situations

Outlining potential problems ... such as a chaotic substance-misusing lifestyle, other drug-using friends and households, procurement of drugs, violence, drug dealing, offending behaviour etc which may put the child at risk

The importance of establishing daily routines and making the home safe and secure for the child

Finally, it is important to remember that the majority of pregnant women and parents with substance misuse problems will provide adequate care for their children and most children will remain living with their birth parents.

Pregnancy is a special event in the life of a woman with substance misuse problems and provides professionals with an opportunity to offer treatment and care that might not otherwise be accepted. The philosophy of approach and principles of management should be broadly the same as for any other pregnant woman with special circumstances and needs.

Service providers

Midwives are specially trained in pregnancy, childbirth and postnatal care. They are usually the lead professional for women with 'low risk' pregnancies. The midwife undertakes a *continuous risk assessment* throughout pregnancy and refers to other appropriate medical professionals if they detect deviations from the norm. They also have a significant role in health education and in supporting parents in the transition to parenthood. All pregnant women are allocated a named midwife at booking. This will normally be a midwife attached to their GP surgery.

Obstetricians/Gynaecologists are experts in all aspects of pregnancy and childbirth. Obstetricians have expertise in treating complications of pregnancy and childbirth and offering specialist advice, screening and treatment. Women with a *medium* to *high-risk* pregnancy will have their care managed by an Obstetrician, with midwifery and GP support.

Neonatologists and **Paediatricians** have the responsibility for looking after the medical needs of all babies, including pre-term infants, babies who are ill (for instance with Neonatal Abstinence Syndrome), and babies with congenital abnormalities. They work closely with obstetricians, midwives and neonatal nurses to plan and provide care for newborn babies in partnership with the parents.

Health Visitors are nurses who specialise in family and public health and are part of the primary health care team. They work alongside midwives to provide parent education and support during and after pregnancy. At the point when the midwifery care ends (normally 10 days after birth) the Health Visitor takes responsibility for the mother, baby and family and will visit in the immediate postnatal period, then follow-up the child until the age of 5 years. Health Visitors play a key role in supporting families with breastfeeding, postnatal depression, diet, exercise, child health and development, disease prevention, parenting, behaviour management, social and emotional issues. Health Visitors visit pregnant women before they give birth and get involved in their care at an early stage. Health Visitors will soon be changing their title to **Public Health Nurse** in line with a move towards working with communities and groups to build their confidence in managing their own health.

General Practitioners have the responsibility for providing general medical care to the whole family and in most circumstances will confirm the pregnancy. GPs are experienced in caring for pregnant women and work closely with Community

Midwives. Many jointly manage *antenatal care* in Primary Care Health Centres. They also work closely with obstetricians and midwives in providing care to women with 'high risk' pregnancies. GPs provide postnatal care to both mother and baby and work closely with Health Visitors. Many jointly manage *baby clinics* with Health Visitors to monitor the health and development of children. General Practitioner's will normally refer the pregnant woman to the community midwifery team and should provide details of any *substance misuse, prescribed drugs* or other *risk factors* on the referral letter or 'antenatal liaison card'.

Pharmacists work in partnership with patients, doctors and other health care professionals to ensure medicines are used safely and to best effect. Community pharmacists are easily accessible to pregnant women. Many are in frequent contact with pregnant women who are drug dependent (especially those on prescription medicines), so can provide support and health care advice. Pharmacists provide a wide range of services including: dispensing of 'substitute' prescriptions, supervised self-administration of methadone, needle exchange schemes and general health promotion advice.

Link Midwives and Nurses (Substance Misuse)

This is a Lothian initiative to improve liaisons in the absence of specialist midwives.

The **role and remit** of the Link Midwife (Substance Misuse) should be:
- To support other midwives within their area to provide good quality care to women with significant problems related to alcohol and drugs
- To promote the implementation and use of the *Substance Misuse in Pregnancy* book throughout the country
- To be a point of contact for other professionals involved in the care of substance-misusing women, offering information and advice where possible
- To liaise with *Link Health Visitors for Substance Misuse,* and other specialist drug and alcohol workers in their area
- To ensure all the midwives in their area use the substance misuse *liaison forms* and collate them for data collection purposes
- To attend regular meetings of the *Link Midwives* and keep up-to-date with trends, research findings, policy and good practice in relation to drug use (including alcohol and tobacco) in pregnancy.

Link Health Visitors (Substance Misuse)

This is, again, a system specific to Lothian.

The **role and remit** of the Link Health Visitor (Substance Misuse) should be:

- To support other Health Visitors within their area to provide good quality care to children and families affected by substance misuse problems
- To promote the implementation and use of the *Substance Misuse in Pregnancy* resource pack throughout the whole of the UK
- To be a point of contact for other professionals involved in the care of pregnant women, children and families affected by substance misuse
- To liaise with *Link Midwives* and specialist drug and alcohol service providers in their area to ensure channels of communication and referral are kept open
- To attend regular meetings of the *Link Health Visitors* and keep up-to-date with trends, research findings, policy and good practice in relation to substance misuse and child health.

References

Abel E.L. (1998) *Foetal Alcohol Syndrome*, Plenum Press, New York.

ACMD (Advisory Council on the Misuse of Drugs) 2003 Report *Hidden Harm: Responding to the needs of children of problem drug users*, Home Office, London. Download from www.drugs.gov.uk

Alcohol Concern (1997) *Brief Intervention*, Factsheet www.alcoholconcern.org.uk

British HIV Association (BHIVA) 2001, 'Guidelines for the management of HIV infection in pregnant women and the prevention of mother-to-child transmission', *HIV Medicine*, 2: 314–334. www.bhiva.org

British HIV Association (BHIVA) 2005, 'Guidelines for the management of HIV infection in pregnant women and the prevention of mother-to-child transmission', www.bhiva.org

Bradley K.A. et al (1998) 'Alcohol Screening questionnaires in women: A Critical Review' *JAMA*, 280(2): 166–71.

Burns E.C. et al (1996) 'The Health and development of children whose mothers are on methadone maintenance', *Child Abuse Review*, 5: 113–122.

Chang G. et al (1999) 'Brief intervention for alcohol use in pregnancy: A randomised trial', *Addiction*, 94(10): 1499–1508.

Confidential Enquiry into Maternal and Child Health (CEMACH 2004), *Why Mothers Die 2000–2002*, 6th report, www.cemach.org.uk/publications.htm

Coghlan D., Milner M., Clarke T., Lambert I., McDermott C., McNally, Beckett M. and Matthews T. (1999) 'Neonatal Abstinence Syndrome', *Irish Medical Journal*, 92 (1).

Department of Health (1999) *Drug Misuse and Dependence: Guidelines on Clinical Management*, Annex 5 'Pregnancy and Neonatal care'. www.doh.gov.uk/

Department of Health (2004) *Children in Need and Blood-borne Viruses: HIV and Hepatitis*, Crown copyright, www.dh.gov.uk/publications

Department of Health (2004) *National Service Framework for Children, Young People and Maternity Services: Maternity Service*, Crown copyright, www.dh.gov.uk/publications

Department of Health (2004) *HIV and Infant Feeding*, Guidance from the UK Chief Medical Officer's. www.doh.gov.uk/

Doberczak T.M., Kandall S.R. and Wilets I. (1991) 'Neonatal opiate abstinence syndrome in term and preterm infants', *Journal of Paediatrics*, Vol.118 (6): 933–37.

Drug Misuse Statistics Scotland (2002) *Scottish Drug Misuse Database*, ISD, Edinburgh. www.drugmisuse.isdscotland.org

D'Souza, S.W, Sugumar, K. Sims, D.G., Miles, J. and Macrory, F (2004) *Methadone exposed newborn infants: Improved overall management resulting from alterations to a service for mothers and infants*, University of Manchester, Academic Unit of Child Health, St Mary's Hospital for Women and Children, forthcoming.

Edinburgh and the Lothian's Child Protection Committee (November 2002) *Inter-agency Child Protection Guidelines*.

Effective Interventions Unit (2002) *Integrated Care for Drug Users*, Scottish Executive, Edinburgh. www.drugmisuse.isdscotland.org/eiu/eiu.htm

Fischer, G. and Peternell, A. (1999) 'The use of Buprenorphine in pregnancy', *Research and Clinical Forums*, Vol 21(3): 17–28.

Ford C., and Hepburn M. (1997) 'Caring for the pregnant drug user' in Beaumont B. (ed) 1997, *Care of Drug Users in General Practice: A Harm-minimization approach*, Radcliffe Medical Press, Oxon.

HEBS (Health Education Board for Scotland) 2003, 'Alcohol – Safe in Pregnancy?' in *Ready Steady Baby* book. www.hebs.scot.nhs.uk/readysteadybaby/pregnancy/health.htm

Hepburn M. (1996) 'Drug Use in Pregnancy: Sex, Drugs and Facts'n'Fiction', *Druglink*, July/August issue.

ISDD (Institute for the Study of Drug Dependence) 1999, *Drug Abuse Briefing*, 7th edition, London. www.drugscope.org.uk

Johnstone F. (1998) 'Pregnant Drug Users' in Robertson, J.R. (ed) *Management of Drug Users in the Community: A Practical Handbook*, Arnold, London.

Kandall S.R., Doberczak T.M., Jantunen M., and Stein J. (1999) 'The methadone maintained pregnancy', *Clinics in Perinatology*, 26: 173–183.

Klee H., Jackson M., and Lewis S. (2002) *Drug Misuse and Motherhood*, Routledge, London.

Koren G. et al (1989) 'Bias against the null hypothesis: the reproductive hazards of cocaine', *Lancet*, 2 (8677): 1440–1442.

Lothian Primary Care NHS Trust (2003) *Managing Drug Users in General Practice*, 4th edition, Edinburgh.

Macrory F., and Crosby S. (1995) 'Special Care or Segregation?: The need for improvement in the provision of maternity services for drug-using women', paper presented at the *6th International Conference on the Reduction of Drug Related Harm*, Florence, Italy.

McIntosh C. (2001) *The Care of Pregnant Drug and Alcohol Misusers in Lothian*, Directorate of Public Health, Lothian Health, Edinburgh.

Morrison C. (1999) in Siney C. (ed) *Pregnancy and Drug Misuse*, Books for Midwives Press, Cheshire.

Mounteney J. (1999) *Drugs pregnancy and Childcare: A Guide for Professionals*, ISDD, London.

NICE (National Institute for Clinical Excellence) March 2002, *Guidance on the use of nicotine replacement therapy (NRT) and bupropion for smoking cessation*, www.nice.org.uk accessed on 1 June 2003.

National Collaborating Centre for Women's and Children's Health commissioned by NICE (October 2003), *Antenatal Care: Routine Health for the Healthy Pregnant Woman*, RCOB Press, London.

Plant M. (1997) *Women and Alcohol: A contemporary and historical perspective*, Free Association Books, London.

Plant M. (2001) *FAS Info: Drinking in Pregnancy*, http://fas-info.uwe.ac.uk accessed on 5th April 2003.

Robertson J.R. (ed) (1998) *Management of Drug Users in the Community: A Practical Handbook*, Arnold, London.

Ross A., Raab G., Mok J., Gilkinson S., Hamilton B., and Johnstone F. (1995) 'Maternal HIV infection, Drug Use, and Growth of uninfected children in their first 3 years', *Arch Dis Child.* 73(6): 490–495.

Royal College of Midwives (1997) *Domestic Abuse in Pregnancy*, Position Statement No.19, RCM, London, www.rcm.org.uk/

Royal College of Midwives (2004) *Infant Feeding*, Position Statement No. 5, RCM, London, www.rcm.org.uk/

SCIEH (Scottish Centre for Infection and Environmental Health) 2003, *Weekly Report*, 15th April 2003, Vol.37, No.2003/15. www.show.scot.nhs.uk/scieh/

SCODA/LGDF (1997) *Drug Using Parents: Policy guidelines for inter-agency working*, LDGF.

Scott G. (2003) *Personal Communication*, Consultant Physician, Department of Genito-Urinary Medicine, Royal Infirmary of Edinburgh.

Scottish Executive (2001) *A Framework for Maternity Services in Scotland*, Edinburgh. www.scotland.gov.uk

Scottish Executive (2002) *Plan for Action on Alcohol Problems*, Edinburgh. www.scotland.gov.uk/health/alcoholproblems

Scottish Executive (2003) *Getting Our Priorities Right: Good Practice Guidance for working with Children and Families affected by Substance Misuse*. Download from www.scotland.gov.uk

Scottish Executive (March 2003) *Responding to Domestic Abuse: Guidelines for Health Care Workers in NHS Scotland*. Download from www.scotland.gov.uk

Shaw B. (1999) 'Maternal Drug Use: Consequences for the Child' in Siney C. (ed) *Pregnancy and Drug Misuse*, Books for Midwives Press, Cheshire.

Shaw N.J. and McIvor L. (1994) 'Neonatal abstinence syndrome after maternal methadone treatment', *Arch Dis Child*, Vol.71: F203–F205.

SIGN (Scottish Intercollegiate Guidelines Network) Guideline 2003, *The Management of Harmful Drinking and Alcohol Dependence in Primary Care: A National Clinical Guideline*, Scottish Intercollegiate Guidelines Network. www.sign.ac.uk

SIGN (Scottish Intercollegiate Guidelines Network) Guideline 2003 *Postnatal Depression and Puerperal Psychosis*, Scottish Intercollegiate Guidelines Network. www.sign.ac.uk

Siney C. (ed) (1999) *Pregnancy and Drug Misuse*, Books for Midwives Press, Cheshire.

Sparey C. and Wilkinshaw S. (1999) in Siney C. (ed) *Pregnancy and Drug Misuse*, Books for Midwives Press, Cheshire.

Stationery Office (2003) *Every Child Matters*, www.everychildmatters.gov.uk/key-documents/

Taylor D.J. (2003) *Alcohol Consumption in Pregnancy*, Guidelines and Audit Sub-Committee of the Royal College of Obstetricians and Gynaecologists. www.rcog.org.uk accessed on 1st June 2003.

Ward J., Mattick R.P., and Hall W. (1998) *Methadone Maintenance Therapy and Other Opioid Replacement Therapies*, Harwood Academic Publishers, New Jersey.

Whittaker A. and McLeod J. (1998) in Robertson J.R. (ed) *Management of Drug Users in the Community: A Practical Handbook'*, Arnold, London.

WHO (World Health Organisation) ((28–30 March 2001) *The Optimal Duration of Exclusive Breastfeeding: Report of an expert consultation'*, Geneva, Switzerland. www.who.int/en/

World Health Organisation (1997) cited in Mounteney J. (1999) *Drugs Pregnancy and Childcare: A Guide for Professionals*, ISDD, London.

Wright A. and Walker J. (2001) 'Drugs of Abuse in Pregnancy', *Best Practice and Research Clinical Obstetrics and Gynaecology*, Vol. 15, No. 6: 987–998.

Glossary

Antenatal care: care provided by professionals during pregnancy in order to detect, predict, prevent and manage problems in the woman or her unborn child.

APGAR score: score measured at birth by observations of the babies health e.g. colour, tone, heart rate etc.

Benzodiazepines: a class of drugs previously called 'minor tranquillisers' which reduce anxiety and have a sedative effect.

Binge drinking: excessive amount of alcohol taken on any one occasion, usually twice the recommended daily amount (i.e. 6 units or more for women).

Bio-physical profile assessment: use of ultrasound scanning to assess foetal well-being.

Birth plan: a written record of a woman's preferences for her care during pregnancy, labour and childbirth.

Brief intervention: usually consists of a brief assessment of substance use, information and advice on risks associated with substance use and details of local services and other helpful resources.

Caesarean Section: an operation where the baby is delivered through an incision through the abdomen and uterus.

Care Pathways: structured multidisciplinary care plans which detail essential steps in the treatment and care of patients with a specific illness or condition.

Child Protection Case Conference: a multi-disciplinary meeting convened by Social Work to assess the level of risk to children and to decide on what action needs to be taken, if any.

CNS depressant: a drug which acts on the central nervous system to suppress neural activity in the brain e.g. opioids and benzodiazepines.

CNS stimulant: a drug which acts on the central nervous system to increase neural activity in the brain e.g. amphetamines, cocaine, nicotine.

Conception: the act of becoming pregnant.

Congenital abnormalities: an anomaly present at birth.

Continuity of care: a situation where all professionals involved in delivery of care share common ways of working and a common philosophy so that the woman does not experience conflicting experience or advice.

Detoxification: process by which a user withdraws from the effects of alcohol or drugs over a short period of time (i.e. 1 to 3 weeks), usually managed with medication.

Deprivation category: the Carstairs and Morris index is composed of 4 indicators judged to represent material disadvantage in the population. These include: overcrowding, male unemployment, social class 4 or 5 and no car.

Drug/ Alcohol Dependence: a syndrome characterised by a cluster of signs and symptoms including physical dependence (e.g. tolerance and withdrawal) and psychological dependence (e.g. compulsion, avoidance behaviour, disregard for harm).

Drug/ Alcohol related problem: refers to a whole spectrum of harm (physical, psychological, social) associated with substance use.

Foetal: of the foetus or unborn child.

Gestation: age of foetus since conception.

'High Risk' pregnancy: pregnancy with increased likelihood of complications, usually managed by obstetrician.

Harmful drinking: levels of drinking which cause physical or psychological harm

Injecting paraphernalia: all the equipment used for injecting drugs e.g. spoon, filter etc

Intoxication: a state where the individual has drunk or taken drugs sufficient to significantly impair functions such as speech, thinking, or ability to walk or drive.

Intrapartum care: care provided during labour and childbirth.

Intrauterine growth restriction (IUGR): previously known as intrauterine growth retardation.

In-utero: in the uterus or womb, unborn.

Lead professional: the professional who will give a substantial part of the care personally and who is responsible for ensuring that the woman has access to care from other professionals as appropriate.

LHCC: Local Health Care Co-operative, soon to be replaced by 'Community Health Partnerships'.

'Low risk' pregnancy: normal pregnancy with few anticipated complications, usually managed by midwife

Midwifery team: a small team of midwives (normally based in the community) who share responsibility for care during pregnancy, childbirth and the postnatal period.

Neonatal period: first 28 days of a baby's life.

Obstetric: the branch of medicine and surgery that deals with pregnancy and childbirth.

Opiates: drugs derived from the opium poppy e.g. morphine, codeine.

Opioids: includes both opiates and their synthetic analogues e.g. methadone, dihydrocodeine, pethidine.

Parity: the number of maternities to a woman (children born live or stillbirth after 24 weeks gestation).

Postnatal: after the birth.

Postpartum care: care provided in the period following delivery.

Polydrug use: the use of more than one drug at a time.

Pre-term: premature baby born before 37 weeks gestation (a 'full-term' pregnancy lasts 40 weeks).

Problem drug/ alcohol use: tends to refer to drug use (dependent or recreational) which causes social, financial, health or legal problems.

Recreational drug use: the occasional use of drugs for pleasure or leisure.

Reproductive health: health of the organs involved in the process of conception, pregnancy and childbirth.

Resuscitation: revival of someone who is in cardiac or respiratory failure or shock.

Screening: mass examination of the population to detect specific illnesses or conditions.

Shared care: an agreed arrangement between a GP and an obstetrician/midwife/paediatrician/or other health specialist over care for a woman.

Social Inclusion: ensuring that everyone regardless of sex, wealth, race, religion, age, lifestyle and geographical position has the opportunity to live full and active lives free from injustice, discrimination and poverty.

Stillbirth: baby born dead after 24 completed weeks of pregnancy. Stillbirths must be registered and the cause of death established before a certificate of stillbirth can be issued and a burial take place.

Substance misuse: taken to mean the use of drugs or alcohol in a socially unacceptable, hazardous or harmful way.

Teratogenic: causing foetal malformations or congenital birth defects.

Tolerance: higher doses of drug are needed to maintain the same effect.

Trimester: each period of three months in pregnancy (1st, 2nd and 3rd trimesters).

Ultrasound scan: image created by use of sound waves, which can confirm pregnancy and determine foetal size and well-being.

Umbilical artery Doppler: is a foetal monitoring assessment test.

Vertical transmission: transmission from mother to baby either in utero, during childbirth or through breastfeeding.

Viral load: the amount of virus circulating in the blood.

Volatile substances: refers to solvents and inhalants including aerosols.

Withdrawal: the body's reaction to the sudden absence of alcohol or a drug to which it has adapted.

Appendix 1

BLOOD BORNE VIRUSES AND PREGNANCY

HIV, hepatitis B and hepatitis C are all blood borne viruses (BBV) that can be passed from mother-to-baby (vertical transmission).

Antenatal testing for HIV, HBV, HCV

In the UK testing for HIV and Hepatitis B is now part of *routine antenatal screening*. While screening for Hepatitis C is *not* yet routine, it should be offered to those with a history of present, or previous drug use. The aim of testing women in pregnancy is to reduce the likelihood of mother-to-baby transmission and to improve and protect the health of both mother and baby.

All pregnant women receive detailed written information about the antenatal screening tests available. At the *booking appointment* the midwife should discuss the reasons for antenatal screening. The implications, risks and the benefits of each test should be discussed and *informed consent* obtained, before blood is taken. All tests are carried out unless the women specifically requests otherwise.

All *negative* results should be communicated to the woman at her next antenatal appointment and recorded in the woman's *hand held* records with her permission.

If an HIV antibody or Hepatitis B (HBsAg) test is *positive* the virologist reports the results directly to the designated lead Obstetrician or Specialist Midwife responsible for Blood Borne Viruses. Some areas, e.g. Manchester, have a Specialist Midwife in HIV/Sexual Health who then co-ordinates the care. An appointment should be sent to the woman to return to antenatal clinic to be given the results in person, and to have more blood taken for confirmation of her positive result. No positive results should be given either by post, or over the telephone. On the return visit, support, treatment and care are discussed. Issues of confidentiality and how to facilitate disclosure must also be addressed.

HIV (Human Immunodeficiency Virus)

HIV is the virus that causes AIDS (Acquired Immune Deficiency Syndrome). HIV can be passed from mother to baby during pregnancy (intrauterine), childbirth (intrapartum) and through breastfeeding. The risk of transmission is related to maternal health, obstetric factors and infant prematurity.[1] It is thought that the

---

1. BHIVA 2001.

majority of vertical transmission occurs during the intrapartum period and there is a close correlation between maternal viral load and risk of transmission, i.e. the higher the viral load the greater risk of transmission. Breastfeeding is also an important route of transmission. The additional risk of transmission through breastfeeding, over and above the intrauterine and intrapartum contribution, is estimated to be between 7–22 per cent.[2]

Without treatment, the transmission rate is approximately 15–25 per cent. This can be as much as 40 per cent if the maternal viral load is high or is at an advanced stage. Research has shown that the prevalence of HIV among pregnant women in Scotland has increased recently. In 2002, unlinked anonymous testing found a prevalence of 5.8 per 10,000 population.[3] Without treatment, HIV-infected children develop chronic disease and about 20 per cent develop AIDS or die in the first year of life. By the age of 6 years, about 25 per cent will have died and most surviving children will have some illness because of their infection. The long-term picture is unknown, but all children with HIV benefit from early life-prolonging treatment.[4]

The *aim* of the antenatal screening programme is to reduce the number of babies born with HIV and to improve the health of infected women and their babies. Diagnosis in pregnancy means that women can be offered advice, treatment and interventions to reduce the likelihood of mother-to-baby (vertical) transmission of the virus. If appropriate interventions are accepted, the risk of vertical transmission can be reduced to below 2 per cent.[5]

The recommended interventions are set out in the British HIV Association (BHIVA) *Guidelines for the management of HIV infection in pregnant women and the prevention of mother-to-child transmission* (2001), the new guidelines for 2005 will be released by the time this book will go to press and can be downloaded from the BHIVA website.

Interventions include:
- The use of antiretroviral drugs for both mother and baby
- Careful obstetric management during pregnancy and delivery

2. BHIVA 2001.

3. SCIEH 2003.

4. Scottish Executive 2002.

5. BHIVA 2004.

- Delivery by pre-labour caesarean section
- Bottle feeding

An expanded version of the BHIVA guidelines, with an appendix on safety and toxicity data is available on the BHIVA website: www.bhiva.org

Management of HIV positive pregnant women

The care offered to HIV positive pregnant women should be jointly managed by specialists from Midwifery, Obstetrics, HIV, Paediatrics, Primary Care and other services, e.g. social work, drug and HIV services, where appropriate. Health care staff should refer to the agreed *management protocol* and care pathway. The approach to treatment is *individualised*, according to the needs and choices of each mother. Good liaison is required between all professionals to ensure that the pregnancy and birth plan proceed appropriately and that the views and wishes of the woman are respected.

There are several *scenarios* where HIV infection may be identified during pregnancy: through antenatal testing, or when a woman discloses her known status when booking. Women who have been unable to tell their partner or family can also use antenatal testing as an opportunity to disclose their diagnosis. Indeed in this situation they should be encouraged and supported to do so.

Antiretroviral drug therapy (ART) for the mother aims to reduce her viral load to 'undetectable'. ART is given according to the mother's HIV health status. Normally it is avoided in the 1st trimester. If possible, treatment will be deferred until just before the 3rd trimester (20–24 weeks) in order to reduce foetal exposure. Women who become pregnant whilst taking ART that is successfully suppressing viral load, will normally continue with their ART throughout pregnancy.

The recommended *mode of delivery* is also dependent on viral load. Caesarean section(c/s) is recommended if the woman declines treatment during pregnancy, if she presents late, the treatment time is reduced or baseline bloods are not available. Caesarean section is also recommended if the viral load result is >1000 at 36 weeks gestation.

If the viral load is <1000 (ideally <50 copies /ml) at term then vaginal delivery is considered an acceptable choice for the mother. With careful monitoring and stipulations such as:

- Shortened labour
- No instrumental delivery
- No artificial rupture of membranes (ARM)
- No foetal blood sampling (FBS)
- No episiotomy

There should be strict criteria for induction of labour (IOL) and also for augmentation or acceleration of labour. In the event of any delays, there will be a accumulated risk of having to proceed to a c/s. These should all be discussed with the mother in advance.

Practices differ around the country, in Manchester, for instance, the woman is provided with a personal care plan that is additionally copied to the hospital notes, the neonatal unit and to the delivery suite. This contains a summary of the intravenous treatment required in labour and the medication and follow-up required for the baby. The woman is advised to give the plan to the midwife on admission to the labour ward. This is particularly useful in the event of unavoidable admission to another hospital that does not have appropriate protocols in place.

Both The Department of Health (2004) and The Royal College of Midwives (2004) state that breastfeeding should not be recommended. However, if a woman decides to do so against the recommended advice, she should be 'supported' in her decision (view the document at http://bhiva.org/chiva/PDF/2004/HIVinfantSep04.pdf).

They also advise:
- that the maternal viral load be monitored, preferably remaining at an undetectable level
- that women *exclusively* breast feed
- that breast feeding should be terminated at four months with immediate weaning.

However, if a woman decides to breast-feed despite the recommendations against it, a multi-disciplinary meeting should be held to explore her reasons for wanting to breast-feed, and the risks this will pose for the baby's health and future well-being. Depending on maternal viral load at time of delivery it is thought that the transmission rate is increased by 8 per cent.

Support for exclusive breastfeeding does not take into account the HIV medication that is given twice daily – and any other additional medication. It is not known what impact this has on the permeability of the gut. Maternal viral load is also known to be a poor marker of the HIV virus level in breastmilk and currently there is no reliable test available.

Seeking both legal and child protection advice should be considered as there is increasingly a case to protect a third party, i.e. the baby, from a significant exposure to the HIV virus.

Antiretroviral drug therapy (ART) is normally given to the baby for the first 4 weeks. The Lead Paediatrician and the Infectious Diseases Consultant should jointly determine the choice of ART to be prescribed. This will depend on the current maternal viral load and any drug resistance at the time of delivery. The medication MUST be given within six hours of birth and the administration times strictly adhered to. This is to avoid any viral break-through, which ensures maximum benefit to the baby.

In Manchester, for example, the mother is provided with a detailed personal post-natal care plan. The baby must have a two week follow-up appointment in order to monitor for any side effects of the medication.

Most neonates born to mothers known to have HIV will be exposed to ART *in utero*. The possible adverse effects of ART to the foetus and developing child continue to be monitored. All women who receive ART in pregnancy are registered with the International Drug Registry and exposed infants are followed up for at least 1 year. To date, no increased risk of birth defects or growth problems have been documented with AZT. However, much less is known about the safety of other anti-HIV drugs. All babies who have been exposed to ART are reported to the British Paediatric Surveillance Unit.

There is an increasing responsibility under the Children's Act (1989) to ensure that a baby born to an HIV positive mother receives treatment, particularly when a parent refuses to agree to this. This may result in the baby being removed by Social Services and cared for by foster parents for the duration of the treatment and to ensure that the baby receives appropriate follow-up. When a woman declines treatment for herself and her baby, a multi-disciplinary case-planning meeting should be held. This must include Social Services. There must be a co-ordinated approach to explore the complexities of the situation with the parents so that they fully understand the potential implications of their decisions.

All babies born to mothers infected with HIV will test HIV-antibody positive at birth due to the presence of *maternal* HIV antibodies. Babies who are not infected will test HIV antibody negative by 18 months of age. Laboratory tests are becoming increasingly sophisticated and can now confirm diagnosis in babies by the age of three months. In Manchester and other centres, the babies are tested at two days, at six weeks and at four months.

All professionals supporting HIV infected pregnant women should be aware of the *psychosocial* issues that can impact on HIV treatment and care.[6] Many women will need considerable help and support to come to terms with the implications of their diagnosis and the management of their infection.

A positive HIV diagnosis should only be disclosed on a 'need-to-know' basis, and must be handled discreetly and sensitively. Consent should be obtained before recording any information in the hand-held notes. For a variety of reasons, many women request that their GP and Health Visitor are not informed of their diagnosis. This presents a dilemma for other health professionals who quite rightly consider that a family-focused approach to healthcare is most appropriate.

Women should be reassured that all health professionals are bound by professional and employment guidelines. Any breach of patient confidentiality is taken extremely seriously and will result in disciplinary action.

Hepatitis B (HBV)

Hepatitis B is a virus which affects the liver and is highly infectious. It can be passed from mother to baby during childbirth (approximately 80-90 per cent transmission rate from infectious 'carrier' mothers). People who remain *chronically* infected with hepatitis B (i.e. 'carriers') can remain well for many years and may not know they are infected. Babies who are infected are at risk of developing serious liver disease later in life.

Preventing HBV infection

The high rate of mother-to-baby transmission can be *largely prevented through immunisation.* If the antenatal hepatitis B surface antigen test is positive, a vaccination programme is started at birth to enable the baby to develop immunity

6. BHIVA 2001.

and to have a healthy life. The midwife delivering intrapartum care should notify the paediatrician when labour commences and ensure that the medication for the baby is in stock. Within 12 hours of birth the baby must receive *immunoglobulin* (which neutralises the virus) and the first *vaccine dose* in the postnatal ward. The baby can then be *breast fed* after these are given. The *second* dose of vaccine is given at one month, *third* dose at two months and the *fourth* dose at twelve months. Immunity checks are carried out at fourteen months of age. The GP and Health Visitor must always be informed, as they are responsible for ensuring that the baby completes the immunisation programme.

It is extremely important to trace any potential contacts e.g. sexual partners, children and other household members, so as they can be offered testing and immunisation where appropriate.

Drug use and Hepatitis B

Even though offering Hepatitis B is part of routine antenatal care, it is *good practice* to recommend all women with a *history of injecting drug use* (or a sexual partner with a history of drug use) full screening for HBV in pregnancy (i.e. the *Ab* test in addition to the *Ag* test). Women with no prior infection with HBV can be safely immunised during pregnancy.[7] Current sexual partners and existing children can also be immunised. Hepatitis B and Hepatitis A immunisation is recommended for any Hepatitis C positive or HIV positive woman.[8]

General Practitioners, Midwives, Health Visitors and drug workers are all in a good position to raise the subject of Hepatitis B, and to recommend screening and immunisation. Immunisation can now be easily carried out in General Practice.

Hepatitis C (HCV)

Hepatitis C is a virus which affects the liver and can be passed from mother to baby, either during pregnancy or childbirth, but *not* thought to be transmitted through breast feeding. The transmission rate is thought to be low (below 5 per cent). People who are *chronically* infected with hepatitis C can remain well for many years and may not know they are infected. Babies who are infected through

---

7. Scottish Executive 2003.

8. Scott 2003.

vertical transmission are at increased risk of developing serious liver disease later in life. Unfortunately, there is *no vaccine* currently available for Hepatitis C. Combination therapy drug treatment for hepatitis C (interferon alpha and ribavirin) is *contraindicated* during pregnancy and breastfeeding (because of foetotoxic and teratogenic effects) and in *young babies and children*. As yet, there are no proven interventions to prevent or reduce the risk of vertical transmission (except in the case of co-infection, see below). *Breastfeeding is not contra-indicated* as there is no clear evidence that HCV can be transmitted by this route. While universal screening of all pregnant women is not recommended at the present time, many health professionals consider that it should be included in the antenatal screening programme, to meet the wider public health agenda.

Identifying hepatitis C infection in pregnancy is therefore useful for the following reasons:
- the woman's health can be monitored
- she can be given healthy lifestyle advice, including the importance of avoiding alcohol
- she can be given advice to prevent further risk of exposure
- she can be immunised against hepatitis B and hepatitis A
- she can be given information on infection control in the home and elsewhere
- she can be referred for specialist treatment once the baby is delivered
- the baby receives appropriate paediatric follow-up

It is therefore *good practice* to offer the test to all pregnant women *at risk of HCV infection*.

Risk factors for HCV include:
- History of intravenous drug use, HIV or HBV infection
- Recipients of blood or blood products prior to 1991
- Sexual partner with a history of injecting drug use
- Sexual partner known to have either HIV, HCV or HBV infection
- Unsterile body piercing, tattoos, acupuncture etc
- Unsterile medical or dental procedures abroad

Because testing for HCV during pregnancy is not presently part of routine screening, the midwife should refer the woman to her General Practitioner or other HCV testing site. Mothers found to be HCV positive should be seen regularly by a specialist, whether treatment is considered appropriate at present or not.

The *Children's Liver Disease Foundation* is an organisation that specialises in supporting children with liver disease (www.childliverdisease.org)

Co-infection (HIV & hepatitis)

Co-infection with HIV, HCV and HBV may occur due to shared routes of transmission. As caesarean section reduces mother-to-baby transmission of HCV in mothers co-infected with HIV, it is therefore recommended, even if there is no HIV-related indication. Drug treatment for HIV disease does not affect the transmission of HCV.

Ideally, all women at risk of blood borne viruses should be offered testing *before* they conceive.

Pre-conception advice offered to known HIV positive women who are planning a pregnancy should include a full virology screen. Their medication should also be adjusted to a regime that is non-teratogenic.

Appendix 2

MODEL CARE PATHWAY: SUBSTANCE MISUSE IN PREGNANCY A2

Pre-conception Care ▼	✓ Advice on reproductive health and contraception ✓ Advice on sexual health ✓ Advice on pregnancy care
Confirmation of pregnancy ▼	✓ The Pregnancy Book ✓ Woman to attend GP (e.g. health advice & folic acid) ✓ Refer to Midwifery Team ✓ Arrange scan
12 weeks **Booking appointment** ▲ **MULTIDISCIPLINARY ASSESSMENT** ▼	✓ Follow antenatal 'Care Pathway' ✓ Assessment of drug use (including tobacco and alcohol) ✓ T-ACE (alcohol questionnaire) ✓ Antenatal Liaison Form (Substance Misuse) ✓ Leaflet 'Pregnant... and using alcohol or drugs?' ✓ Refer to drug/alcohol specialist ✓ Blood Borne Virus testing – if positive, follow agreed protocol ✓ Risk assessment ✓ Commence 'infant feeding' checklist ✓ Consent form for multidisciplinary/ multi-agency working ✓ If woman does not attend booking – follow-up by Midwife

16 weeks	**Antenatal appointment** **IMPLEMENT CARE PLAN**	✓ Discuss and agree care plan ✓ Discuss and agree management of drug/alcohol use ✓ Identify 'lead professional'/'care co-ordinator' ✓ Give handheld records
22 weeks	**Antenatal appointment**	✓ Monitor drug/alcohol use ✓ Monitor progress of care
28 weeks	**Antenatal appointment** **REVIEW CARE PLAN**	✓ Case discussion/care plan review meeting ✓ Reassess social circumstances/risk ✓ Discuss breastfeeding ✓ Growth scan/foetal monitoring
32 weeks	**Antenatal appointment**	✓ Start preparation for parenthood ✓ Discuss birth plan ✓ Discuss NAS and give parent information leaflet ✓ Child protection case conference (if needed)
36 weeks	**Antenatal appointment**	✓ Preparation for parenthood ✓ Assess foetal growth ✓ Discuss labour and delivery (include protocol re prescription)
38 weeks	**Antenatal appointment**	✓ Preparation for parenthood ✓ Monitor drug/alcohol use – update antenatal liaison form

| Term...
(40 weeks) | **Childbirth** | ✓ Pregnancy outcome liaison form
✓ Neonatal Abstinence Syndrome (NAS) assessment and care
✓ Discharge plan (include prescription arrangements)
✓ Discharge pack – discuss info on SIDS (cot death)
✓ Follow postnatal 'Care Pathway' |

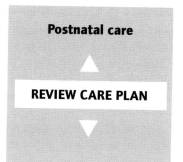

| 10 days | **Postnatal care**

▲
REVIEW CARE PLAN
▼ | ✓ Continue multidisciplinary support/postnatal care plan
✓ Continue NAS assessment and care (if required)
✓ Monitor drug/alcohol use
✓ Relapse prevention support
✓ Midwife ends care (day 10 to 28)
✓ Home visit by Health Visitor |

Appendix 3

CONSENT FORM FOR MULTI-DISCIPLINARY/ MULTI-AGENCY WORKING A3

Please read the following information before you sign this form.

A number of different professionals and organisations may be involved in your care. To provide you with the best possible care and support we need to work together.

Normally we find it useful to share relevant information with each other and to ask each other for advice when we need it. We also need to agree a common 'care plan' with you and keep each other informed about the progress you are making. We also want to make sure that we don't duplicate each others work, give you conflicting advice, or miss out on providing you with something that you might need.

Each different organisation has its own policy on confidentiality and keeps separate written records. Confidentiality can only be breached in exceptional circumstances so we need your consent before we can pass information to professionals who work in other organisations. If you complete this form you will be giving us permission to do this.

I give my permission for the following professionals and organisations to share information regarding my care.

Name: _____

Organisation: _____

Name: _____

Organisation: _____

Name: _____

Organisation: _____

Name: _____

Organisation: _____

Name: _____

Organisation: _____

Name of client: _____

Address: _____

_____

_____

Date of Birth: _____

Signature: _____

Date consent form signed

Appendix 4

NAME AND ADDRESS OF LOCAL HEALTH SERVICE

Date:

Dear Sir/Madam,

I am having difficulty in registering with a doctor.
Could you please allocate me a GP as soon as possible.

I have detailed my particulars below.

Name: _____

Address: _____

_____

_____

Date of Birth: _____

Place of Birth: _____

Last GP: _____

Address: _____

_____

_____

Thank you.

Yours sincerely,

Appendix 5

ANTENATAL SCREENING QUESTIONNAIRE
Alcohol use in pregnancy

T-ACE

T **(tolerance)**	How many drinks does it take to make you feel high? *Answer: '3 drinks or more' scores 2 points*
A **(annoyance)**	Have people annoyed you by criticising your drinking? *Answer: 'Yes' scores 1 point*
C **(cut down)**	Have you ever felt you ought to cut down your drinking? *Answer: 'Yes' scores 1 point*
E **(eye-opener)**	Have you ever had a drink first thing in the morning to steady your nerves or to get rid of a hangover? *Answer: 'Yes' scores 1 point*

Total Score [ ]   Date of test

Lowest score possible = 0
Highest score possible = 5

A total score of two points or more will correctly identify most women whose drinking is hazardous, harmful or dependent.

See guidance on how to respond in *Substance Misuse in Pregnancy: A Resource Book for Professionals*.

Appendix 6

Do you drink alcoholic beverages?
If you do, please take our TWEAK Test

TWEAK

T	**Tolerance:** How many drinks does it take to make you feel high? (Record number of drinks) *Score 2 points if she reports 3 or more drinks to feel the effects of alcohol.* **Score:** ☐	**Number of drinks** ☐
W	**Worry:** Have close friends or relatives worried or complained about your drinking in the past year? *Score 2 points for a positive "yes".* **Score:** ☐	**Yes** ☐ **No** ☐
E	**Eye-Opener:** Do you sometimes have a drink in the morning when you first get up? *Score 1 point for a positive "yes".* **Score:** ☐	**Yes** ☐ **No** ☐
A	**Amnesia (Blackouts):** Has a friend or family member ever told you about things you said or did while you were drinking that you could not remember? *Score 1 point for a positive "yes".* **Score:** ☐	**Yes** ☐ **No** ☐
K (C)	**Cut Down:** Do you sometimes feel the need to cut down on your drinking? *Score 1 point for a positive "yes".* **Score:** ☐	**Yes** ☐ **No** ☐

Total Score ☐

A total score of 2 or more points indicates a likely drinking problem.

Appendix 7

DRUG AND ALCOHOL DIARY A7

Day	Times	Type of drug/ drink taken	Amount taken	Where?	Why?	Effects?

Appendix 8

ANTENATAL LIAISON FORM (SUBSTANCE MISUSE)

Mother's name:

Date of birth:

Address:

Telephone:

Postcode: **Hospital Unit No**

Mother's age: **Mother's Chi No.**

E.D.D: Parity:

                                       Telephone No.

GP:

Midwife:

Health Visitor:

Other drug/alcohol worker:

Social Worker:

Maternity Unit:

Consultant Obstetrician:

Smoker?   Yes/No   If yes, number per day?

Prescribed medication at booking (drugs & dosage)

Dispensing Arrangements?

Pharmacy?   Tel:

Name of Prescriber?   Tel:

Injecting drug use during pregnancy? Yes/No   If yes, please det... frequency

If no, ever injected drugs in the past? Yes/No

Illicit (street) drug use since conception?

(all drugs used, excluding those prescribed, enter average daily amounts taken in 1st trimester)

Heroin	Diazepam/Temazepam
Dihydrocodeine	Other tranquillizers?
Methadone	Amphetamines ('speed')
Other opiates?	Cocaine/Crack
Cannabis	Ecstasy
Solvents/Volatile substances	
Other drug use?	

Referred to **Community Drug and Alcohol Team**?   Yes/No   Attended? Yes/No

Outcome?

Alcohol use (tick average weekly consumption in 1st trimester)?

0–14 units ☐   15–21 units ☐   22–28 units ☐   29–35 units ☐   36–42 units ☐   over 42 units ☐

Pattern of alcohol use? (daily use?, weekend use? binge drinking? etc)

Referred to **Drug and Alcohol Team**?   Yes/No   Attended? Yes/No

Outcome?

History of drug/alcohol misuse in any **previous pregnancies**?   Yes/No

If yes, **outcome** of previous pregnancies?

Additional concerns? (e.g. not registered with GP, homeless, mental health problems, debts, legal problems, literacy problems, relationship difficulties, domestic abuse, sex industry worker etc)

Child care concerns?   Yes/No   Pre-birth child protection case conference held? Yes/No

Antenatal testing for **Blood Borne Viruses**?

HIV test accepted/declined

Hepatitis B test accepted/declined   HBV immunised? Yes/No

Hepatitis C test offered? Yes/No   If yes, accepted/declined?

Referred to **high risk** clinic? Yes/No   If yes, attended? Yes/No

Date of antenatal **case discussion** (around 28th week)

Professionals involved?

Drug/alcohol use of **partner**? (please detail illicit & prescribed drugs taken/alcohol units per wk)

Partner's HIV/hepatitis B/hepatitis C status (if known)

Date form completed:

Signature of key midwife:

Later changes to prescribed drugs? (record any medication/dose changes and date of change)

Completed by:

Photocopy and send to Specialist Midwife

Pregnancy Outcome Form (Substance Misuse)

Mother's name: _____
Baby's name: _____
Address: _____

Mother's d.o.b.: _____

Postcode:
Baby's SM number:
Delivery date:
Gestation:
Birth weight:
Birth length:

Mother's Unit No:
Mother's Chi No.:.
Baby's Chi No.:
APGARs:
Cord pH:
Head Circumference:

Labour ward (please give details (if none state 'none')
Complications in labour?
Pain relief during labour?
Mode of delivery?
Complications of delivery?
Problems at birth?

Postnatal ward
Baby stayed for 72 hours observation? Yes/No
Neonatal withdrawal symptoms developed within 72 hours? Yes/No
If yes, severity Mild/Moderate/Severe
Drug treatment administered?
Medication on discharge?
Breast or bottle feeding on discharge?
Other comments?
Postnatal ward discharge date:
If mother HIV/Hepatitis C positive, baby referred for follow-up? Yes/No   Bloods taken? Yes/No

Neonatal Unit
Admission date:
Reason for admission:
Neonatal withdrawal symptoms? None/Mild/Moderate/Severe

Drug treatment administered?

Medication on discharge?

Breast or bottle feeding on discharge?

Other comments?

Neonatal Unit discharge date:

Toxicology Result:

Community

Baby developed NAS symptoms **after** discharge from hospital? Yes/No

Baby readmitted?

Neonatal Unit

Other please specify

Date of readmission:

Infant feeding at day 10? Breast fed/Bottle fed

Continued drug/alcohol use whilst breast feeding? (please detail)

Date of **postnatal case discussion**:

Professionals involved discussion?

Decisions made?

Child protection case conference held (post birth)? Yes/No

SIDS? (include details)

Age of baby on last midwifery visit?   days old

Date of last midwifery visit?

Name of midwife

Details of Health Visitor

Name:

Address:

Tele.

Form completed by:

Midwifery Team:

Form completed on (date):

Photocopy form and send to Specialist Midwife

Appendix 9

Neonatal Abstinence Syndrome Assessment Score Chart

Unit no:

Name:

Date of birth:

Birth weight:

Gestational age:

	Date:						
	Time:						

SYMPTOM		SCORE						
Feeding	Not able to feed at all	4						
	Demands hourly feeds	2						
	Feeds very slowly (takes more than 30 minutes)	2						
Weight from Day 7 onwards	Loss	4						
	Same	2						
	Gain	0						
Condition of bottom	Raw/broken skin	3						
	Very red	2						
	Mild red	1						
Resting/ sleeping after feeds	Less than 1 hour	5						
	1-2 hours	3						
	2-3 hours	1						
Crying/ irritability	All the time	5						
	Most of the time	4						
	Only some of the time	1						
	TOTAL SCORE							

Drug treatment							
Start time or change dose							

Comments

Please fill in score for each 4 hour period.
Write score for each symptom and add together for total score.
If no symptoms enter score = 0
Insert date at beginning of each day and enter
time at the beginning of each 4 hour period e.g.

23/06
2 pm

Scoring

Mild symptoms = 0-5
Moderate symptoms = 6-13
Severe symptoms = 14-21

Information for parents

If baby has a seizure (fit), dial 999 for an ambulance.
If baby has moderate to severe symptoms, seek advice and help
from your midwife, GP or hospital.

Appendix 10

PREGNANT ... AND USING ALCOHOL AND DRUGS?

Information to help you and your baby

Pregnancy is a very special event for most women. Knowing about tobacco, alcohol and drug use can be important when you are pregnant. This booklet is designed to give you some information and advice to help you and your baby stay as healthy as possible.

Drug use in pregnancy

You may be feeling worried about how your drug use might affect your pregnancy and baby. Most women who use drugs and alcohol have a *normal pregnancy and a perfectly healthy baby*. However, there are risks associated with tobacco, alcohol and drug use.

Unfortunately, good evidence on the effects of drug/alcohol use during pregnancy has been difficult to establish. What we do know however, is that *smoking tobacco in pregnancy* is definitely harmful to your baby and can affect your pregnancy in a number of ways. All mothers who smoke should try to give up! Ask your GP, pharmacist or midwife for help.

Using street drugs (like heroin) or being *dependent* on drugs (like methadone or 'valium') can *increase your chances* of having a *premature birth* and a *low birth weight* (small) baby. This in turn can lead to other problems. The risk of *cot death* is also increased, particularly if you smoke tobacco as well.

There is no good evidence to suggest that illicit (street) drugs alone cause congenital birth defects. Heavy *alcohol* use, however, is associated with birth defects and heavy *cocaine* use is associated with a number of problems in pregnancy because the drug reduces blood flow to the developing baby. Street drugs may contain *impurities* and can put extra strain on your liver and kidneys, so it is better if you can use *only prescribed drugs* when you are pregnant.

It is important to remember that there are *many other things* that can affect your pregnancy at least as much as drugs. For instance, the food you eat (your diet), your social circumstances and lifestyle, and whether or not you get good antenatal (maternity) care. Drug use can affect your appetite, weight, dental health, general health, mood and ability to cope with everyday life.

Changing your drug use when pregnant

If you are using opiate drugs (e.g. methadone, heroin or DF118) try to keep your drug use as *stable* as possible throughout your pregnancy. This means taking the same amount of drug every day and avoiding getting 'stoned' or taking extra, as far as you can.

If you experience morning sickness we normally recommend splitting your daily dose into two lots (one dose in the morning and one at night). Splitting up your dose will keep you and your baby more stable late in pregnancy too.

Injecting drugs carries a lot more risks for you and your baby, especially the risk of infections. It is also associated with premature labour and delivery. If you are injecting drugs you will be given help to stop or cut down if you can. If you are dependent on heroin you will be advised to take *prescribed* opiates instead (e.g. methadone). Seek help from drug services ... they will see you quickly.

Reducing... if you think you could manage to *reduce* your drug use a bit then you would be supported to do so. Talk to your doctor first, so you can do this sensibly. It is important to avoid relapsing when you are reducing, so *slow* reductions are normally recommended. If you are taking benzodiazepines (e.g. 'valium') you will be given help to reduce these first.

Stopping... it is generally safe to stop using tobacco, cannabis ('hash'), amphetamines ('speed'), ecstasy, cocaine or 'crack', solvents ('gas' and 'glue'), 'acid' and other 'designer' drugs. We normally suggest stopping all these drugs in pregnancy. If you cannot stop taking *stimulant* drugs (cocaine/'crack' or 'speed') then get help as soon as you can.

Some women who are *dependent* on opiates or benzodiazepines consider *stopping their drug use altogether*. If you think you might want to do this then you should speak with your doctor or specialist drug worker. *Do not suddenly stop* taking opiates (methadone, DF118, heroin) or benzodiazepines (e.g. valium) as this could be risky for you and your baby. If you want to come off, it is best done under medical supervision, so that your baby can be monitored carefully and you can be given support.

Alcohol... heavy drinking during pregnancy (including 'binge' drinking) is associated with a number of pregnancy complications and birth defects. If you are drinking more than 2 small drinks every day and can't stop or reduce your drinking, then talk to your doctor or midwife who can arrange specialist help. If you are drinking heavily (more than 6 drinks a day) then you should get help straight away. Because we don't really know what is a 'safe' amount to drink in pregnancy we recommend no more than one small drink per day, preferably none.

Drugs and the newborn baby

If you are taking drugs (e.g. opiates and benzodiazepines) most days throughout your pregnancy and right up until the time of birth, your baby will have been exposed to these drugs and may develop *withdrawal symptoms* after birth. It is difficult to predict how each baby will react. It depends on what drugs you have been taking, how much and for how long. It also depends on the baby's ability to clear the drugs from their system.

If your baby does develop withdrawal symptoms, these are usually *easily managed* and the *baby will recover in time.* Sometimes, however, withdrawals can be quite severe and the baby will need special medical and nursing care in hospital (in the 'neonatal unit' or 'special care baby unit'), perhaps for several weeks.

Your baby will be monitored closely for signs of withdrawal for at least the first 3 days and you will be given advice on how to comfort and care for your baby if withdrawal symptoms do develop.

Most babies are well enough to go home after 3 days but may need some special attention from you, the Midwife, Health Visitor and GP for some time afterwards (who will want to check on how well the baby is feeding, sleeping and gaining weight).

Antenatal care (before the birth)

When you are pregnant it is very important that you are checked regularly and attend for all your scans and other tests. Women (and their babies) who get regular antenatal checks tend to do better than those who don't. Midwives are there to help you and will try to answer any questions and fears that you may have. When you see the midwife, let them know about your drug and alcohol use so that you can be offered the special care you and your baby need.

If you have a *drug worker*, tell them you are pregnant so that they can help you with aspects of your drug use during pregnancy. You might also need a *social worker or welfare rights worker* to help with benefits or any other social problem (e.g. housing, debts, legal problems etc).

Normally, the midwife will organise a *meeting* around the 28th week (seven months) of your pregnancy to discuss how things are going and to plan ahead for the arrival of your baby. You (and your partner if you wish) would be asked to meet with professionals involved in your care so that any support that you might need can be arranged well in advance.

HIV, hepatitis B and hepatitis C

Your midwife will offer *routine* testing for HIV and hepatitis B at your antenatal 'booking' appointment. These viral infections can pass from mother to baby. Treatment can now greatly reduce the likelihood of your baby getting these infections so it is important you get tested. If you have *injected* drugs or had *unprotected sex* with anyone who has, you could be at risk of HIV, hepatitis B and hepatitis C. Your midwife or GP will normally offer testing for hepatitis C if you have been at risk. If you are injecting drugs we recommend getting immunised (vaccinated) for hepatitis B as well.

Labour and childbirth

Most women who use drugs or alcohol have a *normal* labour and a *normal* delivery. The obstetrician and paediatrician will get involved if there are any complications. Some women worry about whether or not they will be given enough pain relief ... you don't need to. You will get to take your prescribed drugs *as normal* in hospital *and* you will also be given additional pain relief when you need it. It is important that hospital staff know what drugs you are taking (including any street drugs), as this will affect what pain relief is given (for instance there are some drugs that don't work with methadone, heroin and DF118).

You need to let hospital staff know the name and telephone number of your *pharmacist* (chemist) and prescribing *doctor*. It is *hospital policy* to cancel prescriptions before dispensing drugs in the maternity wards. You should take all your medication into hospital with you and show it to the staff. Be reassured that whilst you stay in hospital your *privacy* will be maintained at all times.

Breastfeeding

You will be given *lots of encouragement and help* to breastfeed, provided your drug use is fairly stable. The *exception* to this would be if you were HIV positive or using large amounts of stimulants (e.g. cocaine/'crack') or street benzodiazepines (e.g. valium) or drinking heavily. Only small amounts of drugs are passed to the baby through breast milk and there is no evidence that hepatitis C is passed to the baby through breastfeeding either. Breastfeeding has *lots of benefits* for the long-term health and development of your baby. If you do successfully breastfeed and continue to take drugs then you will be advised to *slowly wean* the baby onto solids when the time is right. Your Health Visitor will give you advice about this.

Postnatal care (after the birth)

After your baby is born you will be asked to stay in hospital for at least *3 days* (72 hours) so that your baby can be checked for withdrawal symptoms. Following childbirth you might notice that your *normal dose* of drug affects you *more than normal.* This is something to be careful of as over-sedation (nodding off) may mean that you could accidentally drop your baby or not hear them crying.

After you *leave* hospital with your baby, the *midwife* will visit you at home. When your baby is 11 days old, your *health visitor* will visit and will be a good source of information and support on *motherhood* and all aspects of health for you and your baby. There will be *baby clinics* at your local doctor's surgery or health clinic where the development of your child will be assessed. Some areas also have local *parent and child groups* and *breastfeeding support groups* to go to as well.

It is important that you are clear about what is expected of you as a mother and what services are available to help.

The time after the baby is born can be difficult for some mothers. Tiredness and lack of sleep, as well as the 'baby blues' and other stresses (like the baby still having some withdrawal symptoms) can make it harder to look after your baby. This is *normal* and your midwife, health visitor, doctor and drug worker are there to talk to and offer support.

Midwifery care staff

Midwives are specially trained in pregnancy and childbirth. Obstetricians are doctors who care for women in pregnancy and childbirth. Neonatologists are doctors who care for newborn babies. Paediatricians are doctors who care for children. Health Visitors are specially trained in child and family health. All these health professionals, along with your GP of course, may be involved in the care of you and your baby.

Other services

Specialist drug and/or alcohol services may be able to offer you a lot of help whilst you are pregnant and after your baby is born. Ask your doctor or midwife for advice about how to contact them. Specialist services give priority to pregnant women and will see you very quickly.

Some women worry that their baby may be 'taken into care' just because they use drugs. Drug use *in itself* is not a reason to involve the Social Work Department or to *assume* you cannot care for your baby. If there is concern about the *safety or welfare* of your child however, Social Work may need to do an assessment and get involved. This is the same policy for *everyone*, whether or not they use drugs.

Everyone is interested in the well-being of you and your baby and want to make your experience of pregnancy and childbirth a happy one. Please feel free to talk to professionals. They are there to help.

Getting support

It is very important that as many people as possible can offer you support throughout your pregnancy and beyond. Show this leaflet to your partner and any other person (family or friends) who will be supporting you. There are a lot of myths about drug use in pregnancy and a lot of bad feelings towards mothers who use drugs so it is important you get reliable information and have a positive experience.

If your partner also has problems related to drugs or alcohol then they can get help from services at the same time as you, if they are not already doing so. Tell them to speak to the midwife or their GP.

Helpful numbers

Telephone number

My Midwife is

My Obstetrician is

My Maternity Hospital is

My Pharmacist is

My Health Visitor is

My Drug/Alcohol Worker is

My Social Worker is

Other workers involved in my care

Appendix 11

INFORMATION FOR PARENTS

Caring for a baby with drug withdrawal symptoms

This leaflet provides you with information and advice that will help you prepare for the arrival of your baby. Hopefully after reading this, you will feel reassured and confident that your baby can be well cared for and that you can do a lot to help.

If there is anything in this leaflet that you don't understand or would like to talk about further, please speak with your midwife or other health care professional involved in your care.

Drug use and newborn babies

Most drugs (including tobacco and alcohol) that you take when you are pregnant pass through the placenta and are absorbed by your baby.

If a mother is *dependent* (or 'addicted') to certain drugs the *baby* will be born dependent on these too and can develop what is known as *Neonatal Abstinence Syndrome* (NAS). This is a condition where the baby shows signs and symptoms of withdrawal. It occurs often with opiate drugs (e.g. methadone, DF118 or heroin) and benzodiazepine drugs (e.g. valium or temazepam). At birth, the baby's drug supply stops and the baby goes through a period of withdrawal. Baby withdrawal symptoms can be similar to how adults feel when they suddenly stop taking drugs or go 'cold turkey'.

Baby withdrawal symptoms can include things like:
- high-pitched crying
- irritability and restlessness
- tremor (shakiness)
- feeding difficulties (the baby is often keen to feed but cannot suck or swallow properly)
- sleeping difficulties (the baby cannot settle or sleep after a feed)
- vomiting and/or diarrhoea
- fever
- a sore bottom (due to frequent dirty nappies)

Occasionally, babies have convulsions (fits) but this is very rare.

Most babies who have been exposed to drugs before birth will have some symptoms after birth. Some babies experience only mild withdrawal symptoms and require no more than the usual care that all babies need. Other babies however, can have severe symptoms where they cannot feed or sleep properly and they lose weight rather than gain weight. These babies usually need medical treatment, including special nursing care and sometimes calming drugs to help them recover.

Unfortunately, there is no way of telling exactly how a baby will react as there are many different factors that affect withdrawal symptoms in babies. The *amount* of drugs you are taking is only one factor so we like to prepare all parents just in case.

What we can say is that drug withdrawal in babies is now fairly common, so you are not alone. Midwives and other maternity staff as well as Health Visitors and GPs have experience in looking after babies and can offer some good advice and help to parents.

Caring for your baby

Mothers who are dependent on drugs are asked to stay in hospital with their baby for at least 3 days (72 hours). This is because most withdrawal symptoms in babies appear within this time period. Benzodiazepines (e.g. valium and temazepam) however, can take longer to leave the baby's system and withdrawal signs may not show up for a week or so.

In the *postnatal ward* you will be encouraged to *breastfeed* and *'bond'* with your baby. The nurse or midwife will use a special score chart to assess the condition of your baby. You will be shown how to use the chart so you can help the nurses with this.

Most babies are well enough to go home after 3 days where they can be cared for by their parents, with the help and support of the midwife, health visitor and GP. The baby needs to feed well enough and the baby will be checked to see if it is putting on enough weight. Parents are encouraged to keep a close eye on their baby and use the special score chart.

If the baby has severe withdrawal symptoms they would be admitted to the 'neonatal unit' or 'special care baby unit'. Here they can get 'tube' feeds and calming medicine if necessary. Treatment aims to reduce the baby's distress and to get the baby feeding and sleeping as normally as possible. Babies usually stay in the neonatal unit for about 10–14 days, but occasionally for much longer.

Most admissions to the neonatal unit happen when the baby is still in hospital after birth, but babies are also admitted from home if problems become worse later on. If the baby's problems get worse at home then it is better to admit the baby earlier rather than later. This is why we are keen to offer parents extra help at home and to see how the baby is doing.

We appreciate that babies with withdrawal symptoms are difficult to look after and they can require a lot of patience and may be difficult to feed and settle. Some babies can be irritable for months, but symptoms gradually improve with time.

Things parents can do to help

You will have been given this leaflet because your baby may be at risk of developing withdrawal symptoms. Experience has shown us that there are many things that you can do to help calm and comfort your baby.

Here are some suggestions:
- make sure your baby is kept in very quiet and calm surroundings, no bright lights or loud sounds that might upset your baby
- make sure no one smokes near your baby, keep the air fresh but warm
- hold your baby as much as you can, the baby will cry less and feed better if they have 'skin-to-skin' contact
- use a dummy or pacifier ('soothers') ... unless you are breastfeeding
- move and handle your baby very gently; try giving them a gentle massage
- change your baby's clothes frequently, especially if they sweat a lot
- avoid getting your baby too hot
- regularly check and change your baby's nappy
- use a barrier cream around the baby's bottom area to help prevent any skin damage
- feed your baby on demand, frequent small feeds are normally better
- keep a record of all the feeds your baby takes so that the Midwife or Health Visitor can check whether your baby is feeding well enough and putting on enough weight
- if your baby has a convulsion (fit), dial 999 and ask for an ambulance)

Breastfeeding and drug use

All mothers are encouraged to breastfeed their babies and are given help to do so, including mothers who are dependent on drugs. In fact, breastfeeding can sometimes help with your baby's withdrawal symptoms. Only very small amounts of drugs are passed to the baby through breast milk. The benefits of breastfeeding are so great that they outweigh worries about continued drug use. The only exceptions to this would be: if the mother were HIV positive (or 'at risk' of infection whilst breastfeeding); if she were drinking heavily, taking large amounts of stimulant drugs (e.g. cocaine, crack or 'speed') or street benzodiazepines (e.g. valium).

It is important to remember that most women who use drugs have a normal pregnancy, a normal delivery and a normal full term baby. Babies born with drug withdrawal symptoms will recover in time.

We hope that this leaflet has given you enough information to help you prepare for the arrival of your baby. We know that it can be difficult to have a baby with withdrawal symptoms and that many mums feel guilty and 'to blame'. Remember that we are always here to provide you with support and to talk to you about any worries or questions that you may have. Please feel free to speak with your midwife or other health care professional about the information in this leaflet.